ETHICAL ISSUES IN THE NEW GENETICS

Ethical Issues in the New Genetics

Are Genes Us?

Edited by

BRENDA ALMOND
University of Hull, UK

MICHAEL PARKER
Oxford University, UK

ASHGATE

The editors have asserted their moral right under the Copyright, Designs and Patents Act, 1988, to be identified as the editors of this work.

Published by
Ashgate Publishing Limited
Gower House
Croft Road
Aldershot
Hants GU11 3HR
England

Ashgate Publishing Company
Suite 420
101 Cherry Street
Burlington, VT 05401-4405
USA

Ashgate website: http://www.ashgate.com

British Library Cataloguing in Publication Data
  Ethical issues in the new genetics : are genes us?
  1. Genetic engineering – Moral and ethical aspects
  I. Almond, Brenda II. Parker, Michael, 1958-
  174.2'5

Library of Congress Cataloging-in-Publication Data
Ethical issues in the new genetics : are genes us? / edited by Brenda Almond and Michael Parker.
      p. cm.
  Includes bibliographical references.
  ISBN 0-7546-0723-2 (alk. paper)
    1.Genetic engineering--Moral and ethical aspects. I. Almond, Brenda. II. Parker, Michael, 1958 Oct. 6-

QH442.E826 2003
174'.957--dc21

                                        2002190852

ISBN 0 7546 0723 2

Printed and bound by Athenaeum Press, Ltd., Gateshead, Tyne & Wear.

Contents

Notes on the Contributors

Shahrar Ali is Assistant Director of the Philosophy Programme of the University of London School of Advanced Study and Editor of *Philosophy TODAY*, Newsletter of the Society for Applied Philosophy. Prior to embarking upon a philosophical vocation he trained as a biochemical engineer.

Brenda Almond is Emeritus Professor of Philosophy at the University of Hull, England, and author of *Exploring Ethics: A Traveller's Tale*.

Bryan Appleyard is an author and journalist. His previous publications include *Brave New Worlds: Staying Human in the Genetic Future*, and *Understanding the Present: Science and the Soul of Modern Man*.

Robyn Bluhm is a member of the Department of Philosophy at the University of Western Ontario, Canada.

Tom Buller is Assistant Professor in the Philosophy Department at the University of Alaska-Anchorage, USA.

Ruth Chadwick is Director of the Institute of the Environment, Philosophy and Public Policy at Lancaster University, England. Her previous publications include *The Encyclopaedia of Applied Ethics, Ethics, Reproduction and Genetic Control*, and *The Market for Bodily Parts: Kant and Duties to Oneself*.

Walter Glannon is Assistant Professor at the Centre for Applied Ethics, University of British Columbia, Canada. He is author of *Genes and Future People*.

Matti Häyry is Director of the Centre for Professional Ethics at the Univrsity of Central Lancashire in the United Kingdom. He is the author of *Liberal Utilitarianism and Applied Ethics*, and co-author of *Utilitarianism, Human Rights and the Redistribution of Health through Preventive Medical Measures* (with Heta Häyry).

Jonathan Hughes is a Research Fellow in the Department of Government at the University of Manchester, England.

Grégoire Kantardjian teaches philosophy at l'Université de Provence Aix-Marseille, France.

Andy Miah is Lecturer in Media, Bioethics and Cyberculture at the University of Paisley, Scotland.

Ainsley Newson is Post-Doctoral Associate in Clinical Ethics and Genetics at the London IDEAS Genetics Knowledge Park, based in the Medical Ethics Unit at Imperial College London.

Michael Parker is Reader in Medical Ethics at the Ethox Centre, University of Oxford, England. He is a Board Member of the International Association of Bioethics and Associate Editor of the Journal of Medical Ethics. He is author, with Donna Dickenson of the *Cambridge Medical Ethics Workbook*.

Duncan Richter is an Associate Professor in the Department of Psychology and Philosophy, at the Virginia Military Institute, Virginia, USA. He is the author of *The Incoherence of the Moral "Ought"* (Philosophy, no.70, 1994).

Maurice Schouten is based in the Department of Psychology, Vrije Universiteit, Amsterdam, Netherlands.

Tuija Takala is Docent in Practical Philosophy, Department of Moral and Social Philosophy, University of Helsinki, Finland.

Acknowledgements

The origins of this book lie in an international conference organised by the Society of Applied Philosophy at the University of Manchester, in the United Kingdom, which brought together people from a wide range of perspectives to investigate and discuss the nature of the ethical and social challenges posed by developments in genetics and biotechnology, and how they might best be met. We would like to acknowledge the members of the Society and other delegates at the conference for their valuable contribution to the development and genesis of this book.

Two of the chapters included in this volume were previously published in academic journals. We would like to thank editor of the Journal of Medical Ethics for giving permission for the publication of Michael Parker's chapter, 'Public Deliberation and Private Choice in Genetics and Reproduction' which originally appeared in the Journal of Medical Ethics, Vol. 26 (3): 160-166, 2000. And we would also like to thank the editors of Health, Risk and Society for permission to publish Brenda Almond's chapter 'Commodifying Animals: Ethical Issues in Genetic Engineering of Animals' which appeared in Health, Risk and Society, Vol. 2, (1): 95-105, 2000.

Finally, and most importantly, we would like to thank Wayne Williams for the many months of painstaking and dedicated work he has put into the preparation of the final manuscript for publication.

Michael Parker and Brenda Almond

Foreword

Are Genes Us?

Bryan Appleyard

Are Genes Us? No, they are not. Or, perhaps, there is a more precise answer. No, they are not, but they will be if we let them. The first answer – No – is a straightforward denial of the hard reductionism implied by the question. I – and, I hope, you – believe that genes cannot be us because the idea is either scientifically or philosophically unsound. It is scientifically unsound because the evidence we have so far is a long way from being conclusive and much of it is the subject of dispute among scientists. It is philosophically unsound because, first, it presupposes a degree of biological determinism that is at odds with our experience and, secondly, because it assumes a very narrow definition of identity.

In what sense could it possibly be true that a length of DNA is me? It is, of course, not so simple. There are degrees to which we can identify with our DNA or at least with its workings. We might say, for example, that we are 60 per cent genetically determined and 40 per cent environmentally – though how, exactly, we would establish this is open to argument. But it is, I think, clear that, in recent years, those proportions will have shifted significantly in the direction of genetics and away from environment. Not long ago, perhaps in disgusted reaction to the genetic determinism of Nazism, most people would have rated the environmental influence much more highly. Indeed, many people would have claimed that, from the womb to adulthood, we were 100 per cent products of our environment. This was the basis of the desire to improve the world – for, obviously, if you improved the world you also improved people. The increasing precision of the science of genetics has changed all that. Now we know the genetic basis for many diseases and, almost weekly, we hear of the discovery of the genetic 'causes' – I use the word in inverted commas – for many human behaviours from criminality to risk-taking and homosexuality. None of these are firmly based and some – such as the genetic roots of homosexuality – have turned out to be wrong. Nevertheless, the mood of the time has changed in response to this deluge of news from the labs. People now say 'it's in my genes' as casually as they used to say 'it's in the stars' and they read these stories in ways that are similar to the way they read horoscopes – as a form of predestination that has the consoling effect of suggesting their lives are subject to forces beyond their control. More importantly, the claims of new-Darwinism, specifically evolutionary psychology, have been elevated to a potent orthodoxy by the impact of genetics. Once it was seen as intolerably right-wing to claim that our behaviour was biologically determined, now the idea has been enthusiastically embraced by the left.

This brings me to my second answer to the question posed at the start. Our genes will be us if we let them. The genetic determinism that has now entered both popular and academic discourse represents a choice. We are talking ourselves into this belief. Certainly some of the scientific evidence is interesting and some persuasive but none is conclusive. And yet it is being enthusiastically embraced. Indeed, it is being transformed into an ideology, a view of human nature as complete as the Marxist or the Christian. Now, since the questions raised by this new genetic determinism are about identity, the virtues and human nature, they evidently have implications for philosophers. This is their traditional home territory.

At one level the raising of these questions by contemporary science provides occasion for philosophers to engage in debates about the ethical effects of all this. But, at another level, it invades philosophical territory. The truth is that the new genetics is a serious threat to philosophy as an autonomous discipline. Indeed, I fear that the future of philosophy is now threatened by the rhetoric of specifically biological science. Richard Dawkins has predicted – gleefully – that soon theology will no longer be a respectable subject and I think – sadly – that, for similar reasons, the same could be said of philosophy. What will be lost in this process is an ancient and, for me at least, meaningful way of talking about the human experience. It is the urgent task of philosophers to prevent that happening, not only by sitting on committees to discuss reproductive and scientific ethics, but also by insisting on and demonstrating the viability and relevance of the tradition from which they spring.

But first let me explain how I personally arrived at this anxious state of mind. In the 1980's, while writing a book about postwar British culture called *The Pleasures of Peace*, I became aware of a high level of ignorance about science in the arts world. I am not referring here to C.P. Snow's boring old Two Cultures debate. That was a tweedy and entirely parochial spat about a schism within the universities. What I saw was more of an invasion or annexation than a schism. Science was changing not just the world but also minds on fundamental issues. At one level there was technological change, but, at another, there was conceptual change. Physics was addressing issues of origins and even of epistemology. But, more importantly, biology was addressing issues of human nature and values. It is worth noting here that, just after the war, it was a physicist, Erwin Schrodinger, who addressed, in biological terms, the question: 'What is Life?'. That book can now be seen as the moment at which a power shift took place within the sciences, when biology took over from physics and modern science moved decisively into the human realm. Now, obviously, there is nothing intrinsically wrong with scientists asking such questions or pursuing, scientifically, the answers. At the time I simply noticed that it was happening. I noticed, I suspect, because, having had an almost entirely arts-based education and coming from a scientific family, I was aware of what might be called – not strictly accurately – the traditional division between the sciences and the humanities. This division was, in my mind at least, a kind of peace treaty. The sciences described the material world; the humanities did everything else. There was no necessary conflict. But there is now, largely because a number of high profile scientists are no longer willing to admit that there is anything else.

The tendency that I noticed in the eighties accelerated in the nineties. In part, this was a publishing phenomenon. After the success of Stephen Hawking's *A Brief History of Time* with its famous concluding line about 'knowing the mind of God', publishers and scientists wanted to jump on the bandwagon. There was a huge expansion of the sections in bookshops labelled 'Popular Science'. Increasingly this was filled not with physics but with biology and, latterly, with all the areas of science relating to the brain. Books with titles like *How the Mind Works* or *Consciousness Explained* became commonplace. The move from physics to biology and the brain sciences reflected the way that, as Schrodinger had foreseen, life had taken over from the nature of matter and the cosmos as the most pressing scientific issue. This is understandable. Plainly, however much we may be able to say about physics, it would still leave the gaping hole of life and consciousness in the scientific world view. If science was completable, then life had to be part of that completion.

In biology, after the unravelling of the structure of the DNA molecule in 1953, completion seemed to be a possibility. Here was a clear, material basis for life which, at first glance, seemed simple and strikingly reductive in its implications. It seems less simple now. Indeed, I have recently spoken to geneticists who no longer believe that evolution can be the only explanation for the complexities of DNA. But the broad idea that life is a computer-like information system based on the code of DNA is more or less an orthodoxy, largely thanks to the work of highly genocentric writers like Richard Dawkins and Steven Pinker, but also thanks to the media presentation of scientific stories. The mind, however, never looked simple. The pursuit of artificial intelligence has been stalled for decades because nobody can seem to come up with a convincing theory of consciousness, even at the most primitive level. But the deterministic, genocentric orthodoxy was untroubled by that. The mind must be an evolutionary product and it must be explicable in evolutionary terms. Evolution is the one clear self-organising system discovered by science and its adherents have taken on the air of fundamentalists. Nothing, they feel, can stand outside this system because nothing can stand outside science.

The troubling outcome of all this has been what I can only describe as a new contempt for philosophy. My first inkling of this came when I interviewed Stephen Hawking just before the publication of *A Brief History of Time*. He quoted Wittgenstein to the effect that philosophy was now simply a series of language problems. I tried to argue with his interpretation of this but he would not listen. I was shocked. I am no longer shocked by such things. Since then philosophy bashing has become routine. Lewis Wolpert never misses an opportunity to say that philosophers have never said anything worthwhile. And, lately, almost every book I have read on consciousness has paused to lash out at the futility of the work of philosophers. Authors like Pinker and Dawkins, Gerald Edelman, Susan Greenfield routinely assume that current science – brain science in particular – invalidates the thought of philosophers from Plato to Kant and Wittgenstein. The sociologist Charles Murray has gone down a similar road. He has recently written of the near certainty that we would soon find that most human behaviour was genetically determined and this would have radical implications for our political and moral thought. He forecasts, for example, that the left, denied all evidence for its egalitarian beliefs, would be obliged to adopt eugenics as the only way of realising its values. Perhaps the most persuasive and ambitious of these scientists – he is certainly the best writer – is the Harvard biologist Edward O. Wilson. In his recent book *Consilience*, he argued that we were approaching a point at which large areas of human knowledge were about to converge. This convergence would demonstrate a form of completion of the scientific project. Then we would see our true place in the world and we could create what would, in effect, be a new religion. In particular, the insights of evolutionary psychology would show us the correct outline of the good life as predestined for humans by our biological inheritance. This religion, says Wilson, would have the advantage over previous value systems in that it would be true. Philosophy would then, of course, be marginalised as it could only address questions on the fringes of this central and all-encompassing orthodoxy. There is plainly a historical parallel to all this. Galileo threatened the power of the Catholic Church because he showed its Aristotelian and Thomist claims about physics and cosmology were wrong. On these claims, at least, the Church was obliged to back down. Similarly philosophical debates about mind and human identity are now being threatened by genetics and the brain sciences and, it is assumed, in time philosophers will also have to back down. It is all, in the imaginations of Wilson and others, a single process whereby science succeeds in overthrowing first superstition and then all alternative forms of rationality.

How should philosophers respond to all this? Well, they could accept the inevitability of this process. Science did indeed overthrow the church's material conception of the world by showing it was not supported by more technologically advanced observation and by the experimental method. If it is about to do the same to certain philosophical preoccupations, that might be no bad thing. There is no reason why philosophy should sustain itself in ignorance if knowledge is at hand. And it can certainly continue as a cultural and ethical commentary on whatever happens next. Even if scientists explain everything in general terms, it is unlikely they will ever be able to say much in detail at the level of the individual. That leaves a place for the philosophers to interpret their findings in individual cases.

All the same, there are problems with this. First, science has always seemed to be close to completion. Ptolemy was completely right, then Newton was right, then Einstein was right, now maybe Hawking or Gell-Mann is right. At any given moment in history, the prevailing scientific wisdom seems to be unarguable. This is because the cumulative nature of scientific knowledge always gives the present the flattering illusion that it is at the summit of achievement. This may not matter if we are discussing the cosmos. But if, as we are doing now in response to genetics, we adjust our values and most intimate conceptions in the light of current scientific insights, then it is plainly a risky business. What we now know about genetics – a relatively young science, after all – may be radically wrong or dangerously incomplete. Communism was based on bad economics and Nazism, in part at least, on bad biology. But they were not necessarily known to be bad at the time. I suppose this objection is one way of conceptually restating the precautionary principle – we should not do something when we are uncertain of the outcome.

In addition, it seems to me that the very large claims currently being made – notably that we are now on the verge of unravelling the nature of consciousness on the basis of evolution – are patently wrong. In a book called *How the Mind Works*, Steven Pinker admitted half way through that he had not the faintest idea, an admission that prompted myself and other critics to suggest he should be prosecuted under the Trades Descriptions Act. And Daniel Dennett's book *Consciousness Explained* succeeded in explaining precisely nothing and merely said that qualia happened because they would, wouldn't they. Furthermore the huge variation in theories in this area is such that any wise lay person could only reasonably come to the conclusion that we were a very long way from explaining the mind, consciousness or anything else. Even if you think science will one day come up with a convincing account of the mind – and I have my doubts about that as well – then you must still be forced to admit that no such account is on the immediate horizon.

In the mainstream of genetics itself the problems are more serious because they have implications in areas like the law, reproductive decisions, liberty and our whole conception of ourselves as ends rather than means. The more we see ourselves as products of selfish genes, the more likely we are to take radically different decisions about our lives and those of others. Some, notably Edward O. Wilson, would argue that this is not so. They would say that the message of the genes is essentially conservative, that precisely because human culture has evolved the way it has is evidence that human reason would be unwise to overthrow ancient cultural practices. Others have said the same. Francis Fukuyama's last publishing phenomenon was a theory based precisely on this evolutionary conservatism. He argues that the great disruption of the sixties is correcting itself because human nature is driving us back to social rectitude. And Charles Murray believes the revelations of genetics will provide backing for the Republican and Conservative Parties. In other words, we have nothing to fear from this knowledge because it tells us we are doing okay. Again, of course, such arguments depend on the assumption that current science will prove conclusive and, again, I would point out that this is very unlikely to be the case.

But there is another point to be made here. The information coming from genetics is overwhelmingly statistical. In some cases it is not – somebody with the gene for Huntington's Disease is definitely going to get that disease. But, in general and especially in the area of behaviour, genetics is about probabilities derived from very large samples. So, if, in time, we find the genetic basis of heart disease, then we will still only be able to say that any given individual, even with all the high risk genes, has such and such a likelihood of having a heart attack. He may not, for example, smoke or be obese and he may take a lot of exercise, in which case his chances will improve markedly. The importance of this is that it indicates that, however effective genetics becomes, we will always have a wide margin of freedom. The environmental percentage – in which I include the reasoned individual decision – however small it may be, will always be there to ensure that, at the level of the individual, a degree of freedom remains. I remember seeing an item on television about two adult identical twins. One was an obese couch potato, the other was a phenomenally fit and thin marathon runner. They had the same genes, but their choices had produced utterly different outcomes. We will always have a choice and it is unimaginable that any developments in genetics will ever change that.

All of which, I think, answers the question 'Are Genes Us?' with a resounding 'No'. Why, after all, should we decide to abandon our liberty? But I am left with the problem of the persuasiveness of current Neo-Darwinian and genetic rhetoric and its impact on the real, usually irrational world. This impact is increased by the absence of any competing rhetoric. The language of public debate these days is overwhelmingly utilitarian in the most elementary sense. Even the resistance to genetic intervention is couched in the language of the precautionary principle, of possibly harmful outcomes and of risk-benefit analyses. Prince Charles' well-meaning efforts to formulate a spiritual objection indicate how difficult it is to say anything that does not fit into a simple utilitarian calculus. But I believe that there is a competing rhetoric. It is called philosophy. Philosophy has the great advantage that it has been here before many, many times. It knows the territory. Only philosophy can stand outside the immediate terms of current debate and draw attention not to the consoling simplicity of the truth but to its complexity. This is not to say that philosophy should become merely a historical commentary – though it should certainly be that as well. Rather, it is to say that philosophy should find ways of formulating these arguments that do not automatically reduce them to mindless risk-benefit analyses. I know that is asking a lot and I do not really know how it might be done. To say anything at all in these areas that is not marginal or strictly utilitarian is difficult; it implies an entire metaphysical system. But that is not to say that it is impossible. And, crucially, the effort alone is important for, by drawing attention to the freedom and diversity of what goes on in our heads, it makes a mockery of the attempt to apply simple reductionism to the human realm. Philosophy, for me, is a celebration of what cannot be reduced. And it is simple reductionism that is the enemy. This elementary and perfectly sensible scientific technique has, lately as it has in the past, escaped from the laboratory and become an ideology in the world. The writers I have referred to are its evangelists and, frankly, a lot of them do not make sense. They are even more philosophically naïve than me. It is up to philosophers to point this out, even if they are unable themselves to say anything that makes any better sense.

References

Appleyard, B. (1989), *The Pleasures of Peace*, London, Faber & Faber.
Dennett, D. (1991), *Consciousness Explained*, London, Penguin.
Hawking, S. (1988), *A Brief History of Time*, NY, Bantam Doubleday Dell.
Pinker, S. (1998), *How the Mind Works*, London, Penguin.
Wilson, E. O. (1998), *Consilience*, London, Little, Brown & Co.

Chapter 1

Introduction: New Genetics: the Ethical Background

Brenda Almond

Introduction

One of the most widely heard accusations in debates about new developments in biomedical technology, and microgenetics in particular, is that they have placed the creation, control and shaping of life, both human and non-human, in the hands of human beings - abilities which, until now, most civilizations have regarded as God's prerogative. Even those not committed to a religious perspective may share this point of view, although they may prefer to say that the prerogative that is being assumed by human-beings is that of nature itself. It has to be conceded, then, that in a very literal sense modern science takes over a creational role when, for example, in a laboratory an embryologist injects a sperm into a human egg, bringing into existence an embryo for implantation into a woman's uterus. For, if successful, a unique and non-replicable individual person results who, in the normal course of events, would not have existed at all.

But it is not only creation that is possible. Control and shaping of life takes over from creation when there is alteration of the embryo's genetic structure, either to eliminate disease-bearing genes or, more controversially, to create the 'designer baby' - either of these being what may be described as eugenic goals. The hope is that certain 'undesirable' genes can be eliminated from the human gene pool, but more controversially, some would hope that the technology provides an opportunity to spread or maximise 'desirable' traits. In this case, many people today, who are not necessarily committed to any religious perspective, would say that the prerogative that is being stolen is that of nature itself.

The eugenic goal can also be pursued, however, in a way which does not involve genetic engineering, but is equally controversial: this is when various possible lives (embryos) are examined *in vitro* and a choice is made as to which should be given a chance of life, on whatever grounds - gender, health, absence of inherited disease, etc. - and which should be allowed to perish. Finally, another kind of control occurs when life is postponed, as embryos or gametes kept in deep frozen storage may be selected to begin their life years after their original inception, and possibly after the death of their progenitors.

Developments in technologies affecting human reproduction are generally subject to ethical and legal constraints, so that curbs are set on developments in the human sphere. Where plants and animals are concerned, however, regulation is very much more limited, so that both individual and generational gene alteration has been pursued and developed for use in commerce, agriculture and biomedical research. Nature's only defence here may be its dislike of the hybrid, which means that the natural unaided reproduction of the genetically altered species may be problematic.

Along with some scientists and some ordinary non-philosophical observers, there are moral philosophers who view the new possibilities as good, and would wish to see them pursued vigorously without undue legal restraints, while others warn against the hubris of human beings and, whether for religious or more general moral reasons - whether 'pro-life' or 'pro-nature' - would prefer that they should either cease, or be subject to rigorous political and legal control. In the first category, it is possible to cite the Israeli philosopher David Heyd, who, arguing that we need new definitions of the limits of ethics, writes: 'Humans are self-transcending creatures ... there are no moral constraints (over and above the biological, psychological, and ideological) in that constant human attempt at self-transcendence in genesis decisions' (Heyd, D. *Genethics*, p.16).

On the other side are those who have less confidence in humanity's ability to use its technical advances wisely, as well as those who, for religious or moral reasons, want to draw early and embryonic life under the protection of universal rights.

Both the moral questions and some of the political and legal issues are addressed in this book, which originated in a conference organised by the Society for Applied Philosophy on the theme of the new genetics. The conference coincided quite closely with the final unravelling of one of the greatest mysteries of human existence, the Human Genome itself, which is providing us with more knowledge than we are currently equipped to deal with, and with ethical dilemmas for which we have no precedent.

Amongst the issues considered here are: the extent to which, as we uncover the genetic roots of diseases such as cancer, Alzheimer's Disease, and cystic fibrosis, screening should be undertaken to ensure that only 'healthy' embryos are brought to term. The first case, recently reported in France, of a 'wrongful life' suit, is seen by some as a harbinger of a future scenario in which all children will be conceived artificially, monitored and screened - a 'Brave New World' of scientific eugenics in which we - the people of today - will create our future according to the way we *now* think it ought to be - a possibility that some will welcome, but from which others will turn with a shudder.

The theoretical basis of an ethical response

This suggests that the ethical foundation of either response deserves more reflection than that immediate reaction. Nevertheless, the well-known ethical theories usually appealed to here can yield inconclusive results. A positive response is often associated with a secular utilitarianism, but a different assessment of the outcome in terms of human happiness may well lead to a different conclusion, so that utilitarianism is not inevitably identified with approval of the Brave New World scenario. Kantians, on the other hand, in taking seriously the principle of not using persons solely for other people's ends, will hesitate long over the justification of genetic modification. They could, however, defend the use of embryos in cloning, including 'therapeutic cloning' or stem-cell research, if they deny that early embryos possess personhood in the relevant Kantian sense, or if they are able to find a justification in the welfare of the resulting human being. A third approach, that of Aristotelian or 'virtue' ethics, which is conservative about species, can also produce conflicting ethical conclusions. On the one hand, Aristotelian teleological biology suggests that there is an ideal 'type' - a natural kind - of plant, animal or human being, which is violated by genetic interference. But a less conservative view of species could accept the notion of new species and also welcome modification of individual members of species to enable them to fulfil their natural function better.

The application of ethical theory, then, in pure or unqualified terms, may produce ambivalent results. It is up to individual exponents, therefore, to argue carefully for the application of ethical theory to specific issues. This has been the aim of the various contributors here, and in doing so, they seek to throw light on some of the most contentious issues of our time.

In Parts 1 and 2, the focus is on human genetics, while Part 3 raises some issues concerning the applications of genetic knowledge and know-how in the non-human sphere.

Genetically changing human beings

In Part I, the questions raised by the new possibilities for genetically changing or modifying human beings are discussed from an ethical and practical point of view, with a focus on the embryonic stage of human life. Many of these possibilities are already clinical options for parents and the goals of such modification are generally acknowledged to be ethically sound: both doctors and parents rightly want the best for a future child for which they will, in their different ways, be responsible. But while this is accepted by many people as a justification for seeking to eliminate disease-bearing genes, or not to bring to term a disease-affected embryo, many draw back from broader eugenic goals.

In the following chapter, Ruth Chadwick sets out clearly the scientific possibilities and identifies the ethical questions that need to be answered in each case. Where hereditary genetic disability or disease is concerned, avoidance of passing this on to one's children would, until recently, have only been possible by initiating a pregnancy and testing the fetus at a relatively late stage of development. This would often lead to a painful choice and the possibility of abortion. Taking the route of IVF (in vitro fertilisation) makes it possible to select an unaffected embryo prior to implantation in the womb, a procedure known as preimplantation genetic diagnosis (PGD). There is, however, a step beyond diagnosis: a more general screening process known as preimplantation genetic screening (PGS) which can reveal far more than the presence of a specific genetic tendency. These wider possibilities and the possibility of using these techniques to create particular kinds of people, are discussed in subsequent chapters.

In asking whether there is a cost associated with the choices of genetic enhancements, Ainsley Newson acknowledges that prenatal genetic diagnosis is not without problems from the parental viewpoint: the question is whether it is right or wrong for a parent to exercise such a choice - to opt for procreative autonomy rather than the 'genetic lottery'. Her conclusion is that choice is indeed burdensome, but that the offer of choice may be acceptable provided there is no pressure on parents to take it up.

Tuija Takala, on the other hand, adopts a more cautious approach to the use of genetic diagnosis even for limited medical reasons. She considers the libertarian view that children have a right to an open future, that is, that as many choices as possible should be left open to them when they grow up. She concludes that, while such an argument does not justify genetic intervention on a broad front, it may support enhancement which avoids conditions that are commonly assumed to seriously impede a person's open future.

A rather different kind of interference is envisaged where the issue is creation rather than modification or destruction. The idea of cloning human beings has made such an adverse impact on public opinion that many legislatures have rushed forward legislation to ban it. The accusation of 'playing God' is most frequently heard in this context, and it is in these terms that the issue of cloning is raised by Duncan Richter. He asks whether we should be afraid of 'playing God' by cloning human beings. This is, he concludes, despite reservations, a reasonable fear. However, notwithstanding possible objections from legal conservatives, Richter comes down in the end in favour of the view that cautious and slow progress should be allowed.

His conclusions are shared by the Finnish philosopher Matti Häyry, who discusses a possible objection to cloning based on its offensiveness to people's feelings. Häyry, too, is interested in the legal conservative position associated with the views of the late Lord Devlin, for whom morality, as epitomised in the views of ordinary people and their reactions of disgust or approbation, constitutes the essential cement of a society. However, he argues that 'Devlinian disgust' is not a reason for objecting to such developments.

Walter Glannon's chapter opens up the possibility that the questions raised are not only ethical and practical, but that deep philosophical questions about personal identity and human freedom are raised as well. Are we, perhaps, no more than the sum of our genes? Focussing on the issue of genetic intervention when undertaken for sound medical and therapeutic reasons, Glannon asks whether or to what extent gene therapy affects identity. The answer, he says, depends on the stage of development of the embryo at which intervention takes place. Early genetic interference, he argues, *does* affect identity, since at that stage identity has not yet been formed. But later genetic interference, Glannon believes, does not change identity in the same way, or indeed at all.

Genetics and personal identity

Part II explores this issue of identity on a wider front. Tom Buller discusses the claims of genetic reductionism, the view that a person's health can be determined by their genetic make-up, and whether recent developments in genetics will lead to a revision in our existing theory of health and disease. He argues that although the more strident versions of genetic reductionism appear to be false, there is evidence to suggest that we have already begun to revise our notions of health and disease, and to place greater emphasis on the presence or absence of genetic disease traits and less on the physical and phenomenological aspects of illness. He then asks whether our existing theory will continue to be accommodated by the new theory or will it eventually be replaced.

Robyn Bluhm, too, supports the view that we do not need to end up with deterministic conclusions as a result of the new discoveries that suggest that there may be a genetic basis for factors ranging from illness to intelligence. Although our genes are indeed part of us, she points out that we are also formed by our environment and our culture and this means, she argues, that there is still a role for personal responsibility and for a realistic notion of choice.

Maurice Schouten offers an argument which supports this conclusion, but is based on scientific investigation of a possible genetic component in memory and learning. Referring to the technique of gene targeting that is sometimes used in learning and memory research, Schouten argues that psychological functions cannot be reduced to molecular genetics. He suggests that the contribution of genetic factors is better accounted for by a more complex theory of 'explanatory pluralism' which seeks to analyse the relations between mind, brain, behaviour, and genome. Like Bluhm, he, too, points out that there is also an environmental and cultural context to be taken into account.

Most are agreed that human gametes - sperm and eggs - are the vehicles of genes with varying potential. As a result of this recognition, a market has already grown up in the United States for the gametes, and hence the genes, of people with sought-after characteristics. Andy Miah discusses this, and also the patenting of human DNA. He writes that commercial companies are now seeking to obtain patent rights on some aspects of the human genome. In considering the question of how people's identity relates to their genetic heritage from this point of view, he concludes that patenting and ownership might not be unacceptable in themselves, but that the important issue is the use that is made of this genetic information and of possible further commercial developments, in which the buying and selling of human genetic material and its use for eugenic goals may become routine.

Gregoire Kantardjian, who also considers the ethics of genetic intervention, is specifically interested in this issue of law and regulation. If genes are involved in the constitution of personal identity, he asks, should limits be set to the new genetics? His conclusion is that genetic modification of human beings is not justified, even with consent, since we do not own our bodies, but have only a kind of 'tenancy right' in them. Hence, we have a right to the use, but not the abuse, of our bodies.

Genes and the non-human living world

In Part III, the focus shifts from humans to other aspects of the natural world. Again, there are positive implications. The benefits are often vigorously promoted: superplants to feed Third World communities, 'green' fuels to replace petrol, microbes to purify water, extract minerals from soil, or clear up oil-spills from the ocean. But there are clear signs of a more cautionary approach being applied to these issues.

Brenda Almond argues that the patenting of life in agribusiness and for scientific research involves serious ethical issues which are not confined to the question of risk, but also involve our conception of a species and the view we take of our new ability to move the pace of evolution forward at an unprecedented pace.

Turning to the area of agriculture, Jonathan Hughes suggests that in the case of genetically modified crops, the precautionary principle does not create a sufficiently strong case for a moratorium. He therefore recommends a cautious and creative approach in the interests of promoting progress in the important task of alleviating hunger in the Third World.

Shahrar Ali also considers the assessment of risk in relation to the release of genetically modified organisms and crops but his discussion focusses especially on the needs and expectations of the European countries. He, too, puts the case for cautious advance, but with greater emphasis on the qualitative aspects associated with risks.

In a closing chapter, Michael Parker concludes the debate engaged in by the contributors to the present volume by pointing to some potential directions for future policy. These must, he argues, recognise the fundamental disagreements about these matters that will no doubt continue to make political and legal decision-making difficult and problematic. He suggests, however, that public policy can usefully be founded on recognition of the areas of life in which personal autonomy should rule and of those in which the decisions to be reached are essentially community decisions for which new forms of public consultation and new democratic procedures are appropriate – a process of public debate to which the present book itself seeks to make a contribution.

PART 1

The Genetic Modification and Invention of Human Beings

Chapter 2

Genetic Possibilities

Ruth Chadwick

The completion of the first draft of the human genome has given fresh impetus to debates about genetic possibilities and their applications in medicine, and also about the philosophical and ethical implications. Publication of the results has facilitated predictions of a paradigm shift in medicine (Schmidt, 1998): questions arise concerning not only the extent to which these predictions are sound, but also the need for new thinking in ethics. Genetics has tested the limits of ethical thinking in a number of ways, partly in so far as it has led to discussions of personhood and determinism, and partly in giving rise to re-examination, not only of the applicability, but also of the meaning of concepts such as autonomy and privacy. Further, while a central concern among both bioethicists and the public has been control over genetic data, and while this has usually been discussed in terms familiar from medical ethics – that is, as a right of confidentiality and privacy, for some time debates about 'new genetics' have given rise to vigorous debates over the thesis of genetic exceptionalism. This thesis holds that there is a difference in kind between genetics and other areas of medicine, because, for example, genetic information is predictive, not specific to time, and shared between blood relatives. The difference in kind, if there is one, may also affect the terms in which the ethical debated should be conducted. Arguments against genetic exceptionalism point to other areas of medicine that share, at least to some extent, some of these features: there are non-genetic tests that are predictive; a person's HIV status is relevant not only to him or herself.

It is not my purpose here to try to defend genetic exceptionalism, but I do want to defend the less strong view, that there is a danger that we may be attempting to apply doctrines developed in the 20th century, in response to specific circumstances, to 21st century problems. There are good reasons for taking the view that genetics renders problematic the application of some principles, or at least that some aspects of genetics such as pharmacogenetics and genetic databases do this.

It is increasingly accepted that traditional thinking in ethics *is* challenged by developments in genetics. For example, in *From Chance to Choice* (2000) Allen Buhcanan, Dan Brock, Norman Daniels and Dan Wikler have argued that where distributive justice is concerned, there is a need for a radical rethink. They argue that theories of justice have framed the problem of justice as one of distributing social benefits and burdens between participants in the co-operative framework, but that this overlooks the ways in which the choice of a co-operative framework itself determines who the participants *are*. This is relevant, for example, in relation to some of the criticisms of the new genetics from organisations and individuals concerned with the rights of persons with disabilities. These include the 'loss of support' argument (that it will become more difficult for persons with disabilities to access social support or facilities, because they may be regarded, in the changed situation, as having 'elective disability'); and the 'expressivist' objection (that decisions in favour of genetic intervention express negative judgements about persons with disabilities). Buchanan et al. offer good grounds for the view that such criticisms are misconceived, but acknowledge that there is a danger that the new genetics *is* exclusionary in some sense. Without *reducing* disability to a social construction they recognise the ways in which theories of justice can construct disability and argue that this poses a clear challenge for theories of justice to create co-operative frameworks that are inclusive.

While this is a claim about the 'new genetics' overall, I want to look at one development in genetics that has raised the issue anew and particularly starkly, namely pharmacogenetics and the potential impact of pharmacogenetic testing. 'Pharmacogenetics' is the term used to describe the use of genetic information to show how variations in patients' DNA may affect drug responsiveness and susceptibility to side effects. In the case of a given drug we may know that it will help a certain proportion of people while others will suffer from adverse reactions. Pharmacogenetics will enable us to identify who will be likely to benefit and who harmed, so that prescribing the product to the latter group can be avoided. It affects, potentially, the whole of health care, not only that part which deals with genetic disorders or with genetic susceptibility to common disease; it has implications for both therapy and clinical trials. It raises the issue of genetic exceptionalism anew for several reasons: it has been argued that it will individualise medicine and challenge professional roles and that even as compared with other areas of genetics, the relevant ethical considerations and principles are different (Roses, 2000b). In fact, we might even be tempted to coin the term 'pharmacogenetic exceptionalism'.

John Bell, writing in the *British Medical Journal*, has predicted that pharmacogenetics might lead to a new understanding of disease (Bell, 1998). Whereas common diseases are currently defined by their clinical appearance, it will become possible to subdivide heterogeneous diseases into discrete conditions, in other words, change our perception of what the condition is for which the treatment is sought (Roses, 2000a). As genetic variants are identified that are associated with drug response there is likely to be a move towards widespread testing before prescribing – in fact it may come to be considered unethical not to carry out such tests (Wolf et al., 2000). The type of testing involved, however, is different from testing for single gene disorders: it will involve testing for single nucleotide polymorphisms (SNPs) and thus the transferability of guidelines developed for other kinds of testing cannot be assumed (Roses, 2000b).

Screening and testing

Bell argued that the 'development of drugs along genetic guidelines will be a major force driving the implementation of screening by healthcare providers' (Bell, 1998). If this were the case, then it might be expected that we should turn to the guidelines developed for evaluating screening programmes. The first criterion frequently referred to in discussions of genetic screening, is whether the condition sought is an important health problem, or whether it is 'serious' (e.g., Nuffield Council on Bioethics, 1993). There has been considerable discussion over what counts as serious, but despite the difficulties over a precise definition there is a widespread consensus on particular examples of conditions that are life-threatening, including some of the cancers and the hemoglobinopathies such as thalassemia.

In the case of pharmacogenetic testing of an individual's medicine response profile, however, the 'condition' sought is susceptibility to drug toxicity – in other words, a manufactured or iatrogenic condition. Does this count as an 'important health problem' or 'serious' condition? It might seem so, because it has been estimated that adverse drug reactions account for more than 2 million hospitalisations and 100,000 deaths per annum in the United States (quoted in Schmidt, 1998; Stix, 1998), and these figures have been used to demonstrate the benefits of pharmacogenetics. We cannot use them, however, to justify a pharmacogenetic screening programme in relation to any one condition or treatment. They would be useful if what was sought were a predisposition to find all the drugs implicated in these figures toxic, or some trait that might be applicable across the spectrum, such as being a slow metaboliser. Otherwise we need to have product-specific information.

The second criterion to be discussed concerns what can be done in the light of a positive result. Where what is sought is a genetic diagnosis of an existing or presymptomatic condition, or a prediction of a late onset condition or predisposition, what might be at issue is the availability of treatment. In the case of pharmacogenetics, however, this criterion again has problematic applicability. What is being investigated is the extent to which the treatment itself is potentially toxic for particular individuals, so it is difficult to use availability of treatment as a criterion of screening since the screening is being carried out to establish the extent to which *this* treatment *is* an 'available' treatment.

What may be envisaged, however, is not population wide screening but individual *testing*. Some of the literature on this topic has described developments in pharmacogenetics as facilitating 'personal pills' (Persidis, 1998), the suggestion being that awareness of genetic variation between individuals will facilitate prescribing in accordance with the specific needs of the individual, thus arguably in accordance with a principle that health care resources should be allocated according to need at the point of delivery. Pharmacogenetics has the potential to individualise prescribing by affecting a prescribing decision for a given patient in at least three different ways: (1) adjustment of dosage of drug A; (2) a choice between prescribing drug A or drug B; (3) drug A or nothing (where there is no alternative treatment available). The ethical issues related to monitoring of appropriate dosage as compared with choice of medication need to be considered. The situation where the choice is between drug A and *no* medication gives rise to the ethical problem of perceived or actual abandonment.

A major feature of the debate about the introduction of other genetic screening and testing programmes has been the right to know versus the right not to know question, supported by competing interpretations of concepts such as autonomy and solidarity (cf. Chadwick, Levitt and Shickle, 1997). It has been argued that there might be a right not to know genetic information about, for example, one's future health status – such information may lead to depression, turn out be a self-fulfilling prophecy, affect one's self-image and/or lead to social stigma or other disadvantage. But it might appear that the same considerations would not apply in relation to susceptibility to drug toxicity – surely it could only be beneficial to have information enabling one to avoid the side effects of drugs? This is one possible example of 'pharmacogenetic exceptionalism'. A right to know one's genetic status vis-à-vis susceptibility to drug toxicity might be supported by an autonomy-based argument where autonomy is interpreted in terms of self-determination – facilitating the choice of the individual in relation to treatment. In the event of multiplex testing, however, it might be possible to test at the same time for predisposition to a disease and for susceptibility to toxicity for the standard treatment. Then the question arises as to whether having this information is a benefit or a burden, because this is analogous to the situation where there is *no* treatment available. In such a case the argument for a right not to know comes into play.

Are there any other reasons that might ground a right not to know about susceptibility to drug toxicity? The knowledge that one has a higher risk of toxicity might in itself increase that risk. Further, genetic susceptibility to drug toxicity may have insurance implications in the way that genetic predisposition to health problems might – people slow, because of their genotype, to clear drugs from their bodies, or to convert them to nontoxic form, may be identified as belonging to a higher insurance risk category (Schmidt, 1998).

Connected with this problem is the issue of quality control in a situation where hundreds of thousands of tests are carried out annually. External quality assessment schemes (EQAs) of genetic tests in Europe have demonstrated a low but significant error rate in cystic fibrosis testing (Dequeker et al., 2001) and the number of laboratory tests carried out annually as pharmacogenetic testing comes on stream is set to increase dramatically. Mistakes may arise not only through technical error but also out of clerical error or sample mix-up (Dequeker et al., 2001).

Apart from the possibility of error, there are problems with uncritically accepting that an identification of genetic risk factors will determine or assist in determining the appropriate treatment for a particular patient. Other factors such as food intake, general state of health and age may account for someone's response to a drug (Haseltine, quoted in Stix, 1998; Chadwick and Levitt, 1995); drug efficacy and toxicity may be considered as multifactorial traits that involve some genetic component(s) in much the same way as complex diseases do. Beyond the issues for individuals, patients could be stratified according to genetic risk factors, as they are presently classified by other risk factors such as high blood pressure (Chadwick,

1999; Wolf et al., 2000). In this connection the possible implications for particular population groups should be considered, in the light of possible differences between ethnic groups as regards, for example, slow or rapid rate of metabolising a drug.

Thus patient stratification could have discriminatory implications. One possibility is that genetic susceptibility might be correlated with some other characteristic such as ethnicity, leading in effect to a presumption of effective treatment for that condition for that particular group although there might be considerable variation within the group. The Council on Ethical and Judicial Affairs of the American Medical Association in an article on 'Multiplex genetic testing' in the Hastings Centre Report (1998) argued that;

> ethnic heritage may contribute to particular concerns, it is clinically relevant and should be considered. Offering multiplex tests that are bundled according to race of ethnicity, however, serves to categorise patients rather than to address their distinct needs ... The profession can ill afford the perception that science is being used to bring attention to the genetic flaws present in lines of inheritance. (Council for Ethical and Judicial Affairs, 1998)

Indeed there is some support for the view that the significance of ethnic variation in drug response might have been overstated (Hodgson and Marshall, 1998).

Professional ethics

Questions for professional ethics arise when considering how pharmacogenetics will affect health care delivery. Different modes of delivery will raise different ethical questions, and countries may differ in how they integrate pharmacogenetics into health care. If genetic testing becomes a standard accompaniment of prescribing, there are questions about how this will be carried out. If doctors carry out medicine response testing at the time of prescription then this will 'geneticise' doctor-patient interactions, with all the associated concerns about the potential use, misuse, understanding and misunderstanding of genetic information. There may be, however, a number of other ways in which medicine response profiles could be accessed. One could be a central database, containing patient genotype information, which will be accessed at the time of prescription. If the latter is the case then quality control issues, mentioned above, become particularly important to prevent errors being perpetuated over time. The person who accesses this database, however, need not be the doctor – it may be, for example, the pharmacist. There may be an expanding role here for pharmacists, if for example doctors *prescribe* generically and pharmacists *dispense* according to genotype. There is a need, however, to think through the ethical implications for doctors and pharmacists arising out of these possible changes to their roles. The last scenario may be more appropriate in certain applications of pharmacogenetics, e.g. when the choice is between drug A and drug B.

Changes in professional roles, if the situation develops in this way, suggest a need for education and training in the ethical implications. What form this training should take will depend on how the ethical issues should be addressed, and this is one respect in which challenges to existing ethical frameworks become significant. As already indicated there is specific concern about the transferability of existing guidelines to pharmacogenetics, as suggested by Allen Roses: 'It is ... incumbent that medical guidelines for mendelian- or susceptibility-gene testing do not extend automatically to discussions of other types of genetically based profiles in pharmacogenetics. Clear language and differentiation of respective ethical, legal and societal issues are required...' (Roses, 2000b). Roses, addressing the annual Human Genome Meeting in 2001, argued that privacy concerns may be less acute in pharmacogenetic testing than in testing for single gene disorders or for susceptibility to common diseases. Whether this point should be accepted, however, turns on the extent to which the information could be used to an individual's disadvantage, and some ways in which this might be the case have been noted.

Clinical trials

Clinical trials in this area may have features that distinguish them from traditional clinical trials: first, it should be possible for clinical trials to become more targeted towards specific groups. For present purposes, however, the salient point is that they are likely to involve storage of DNA samples as responses to drugs are tracked over time, and this raises questions about the feasibility of informed consent. In the course of the debates about genetic exceptionalism concerns have been voiced about the possibility of genuine informed consent in genetics generally (cf. Chadwick, 2001) but in the case of long term storage of DNA samples the issues become particularly complex because of the difficulty of making sense of 'consenting' to potential but presently unforeseeable uses of one's samples at some point in the future (cf. Chadwick and Berg, 2001).

The challenge to the applicability of informed consent raised by storage of genetic data arises in connection with pharmacogenetics without being unique to genetic databases used for pharmacogenetic purposes. It does not support, therefore, pharmacogenetic exceptionalism, any more than genetic exceptionalism. It is an important example, however, of how the applicability of traditional ethical frameworks is coming under challenge. Justice, privacy, informed consent, autonomy: these are all subject to reconstrual in the light of developments in genetics. While it might be argued that this is what should be expected in relation to philosophical and ethical concepts in any case, this is not the whole story. The point is that this area of 'applied ethics', in particular, suggests a need to be sensitive to the inappropriateness of a model of *application* which takes pre-existing theories and principles with a view to 'applying' them to (pharmaco)genetics. Rather, we should be open to possibilities not only of 'new genetics' but also of new ways of doing ethics.

References

Bell, J. (1998), 'The new genetics in clinical practice' *British Medical Journal*, vol. 316, pp.618-20.

Buchanan, A., Brock, D.W., Daniels, N. and Wikler, D. (2000), *From Chance to Choice: Genetics and Justice,* Cambridge, Cambridge University Press.

Chadwick, R. (1999), 'Criteria for genetic screening: the impact of pharmaceutical research' *Monash Bioethics Review,* vol. 18, pp.22-6.

Chadwick, R. (2001), 'Informed consent and genetic research', in L.Doyal and J.Tobias (eds) *Informed Consent and Medical Research,* London, BMJ Books.

Chadwick, R. and Berg, K. (2001), 'Solidarity and equity: new ethical frameworks for genetic databases' *Nature Reviews Genetics,* vol. 2 pp.318-21.

Chadwick, R. and Levit, M.A. (1995), 'When Drug Treatment in the Elderly is not cost-effective: An Ethical Dilemma in Environment of Healthcare Rationing', *Drugs and Ageing,* vol. 7(6), pp.416-19.

Chadwick, R., Levitt, M. and Shickle, D. (eds) (1997), *The right to know and the Right not to Know*, Aldershot, Avebury.

Council on Ethical and Judicial Affairs, American Medical Association (1998), 'Multiplex genetic testing' *Hastings Centre Report,* vol. 28(4), pp.15-21.

Dequeker, E. et al., 'Quality control in molecular genetic testing', *Nature Reviews Genetics,* vol. 2(9), pp.717-23.

Hodgson, J. and Marshall, A. (1998), 'Pharmacogenomics: will the regulators approve?' *Nature Biotechnology,* vol. 16, pp.243-6.

Housman, D. and Ledley, F.D. (1998), 'Why pharmacogenomics? Why now?' *Nature Biotechnology,* vol. 16, pp.492-3.

Nuffield Council on Bioethics (1993), *Genetic Screening Ethical Issues,* London, Nuffield Council on Bioethics.

Persidis, A. (1998), 'The business of pharmacogenomics', *Nature Biotechnology,* vol. 16, pp.209-10.

Roses, A.D. (2000a), 'Pharmacogenetics and future drug development and delivery' *The Lancet,* vol. 355, pp.1358-61.

Roses, A.D. (2000b), 'Pharmacogenetics and the practice of medicine' *Nature,* vol. 405, pp.857-65.

Schmidt, K. (1998), 'Just for you' *New Scientist,* vol. 160(2160), pp.32-6.

Stix, G. (1998), 'Personal Pills' *Scientific American,* vol. 279(4), pp.10-11.

Chapter 3

Is There a Cost in the Choice of Genetic Enhancement?[1]

Ainsley Newson

Introduction

In addition to finding 'genes for' genetic disease, genetic researchers are also currently identifying genes involved in the development of behavioural traits such as intelligence. The primary aims of this research are to contribute to the scientific understanding of brain development and to develop interventions to assist those with low intellectual potential. However, this information could potentially also be utilised by parents to choose to have a child with a genetic predisposition to high intelligence.[2] In this chapter, I unpack a potential objection to this technology: that it offers parents a reproductive choice they would be better off without.

Many objections raised against genetic enhancement technology to date are problematic.[3] In justifying enhancement, some authors appeal to the non-identity problem (Parfit, 1984, Ch.16) to claim that from the affected child's perspective, there can be no objection to genetic intervention before birth unless the resulting child's life is so bad that it is not worth living (see, e.g.: Harris, 1997; Harris, 1998a; Robertson, 1994). This sets a very high standard of harm to justify a prevention of genetic intervention, and does not seem to explain the intuitive response most people have to the idea of genetic enhancement technology. By altering the focus of ethical investigation from examining outcomes for individuals born from enhancement procedures, to instead examining the acts of parents in choosing to use this technology, this paper presents a potential way to re-negotiate such problems with procreative autonomy.

Practitioners of clinical genetics place substantial value upon individual choice, yet to date very little discussion has taken place as to whether exercising an expanded amount of procreative autonomy could ever carry a cost for parents. Consider the following scenario:

> Tom and Jane are carriers of a genetic disease. In order to avoid having to undergo pre-natal diagnosis and potentially face a termination decision, they opt to undergo pre-implantation genetic diagnosis and IVF.

Of six embryos, two are affected and four are not. Their doctor then asks them if they would like to know the potential intelligence of the four unaffected embryos.

Is this a choice that Tom and Jane are going to want to have?

Making the choice to select for intelligence may carry a number of unique costs, which I identify and evaluate in this chapter. To do this, I first discuss the value of having choices generally. I then consider several costs that could detrimentally affect parents' interests in choosing the intelligence of their child.

I argue that having choices in procreation is generally valuable for parents as it promotes individual freedom and autonomy. However, I also argue that giving parents 'genetic enhancement choices' will only be good if it increases the total range of desirable options that they have. In then analysing whether or not genetic enhancement presents a desirable option for parents, I claim that these choices may carry some costs, but that these are not significant enough to warrant overriding procreative autonomy. However, it is still important to identify these costs, as it will be essential to convey the potential problems of genetic enhancement choices to parents during the process of obtaining informed consent.

What is the value of having choices?

C. Mills writes: 'We want to believe that the central facts of our lives... contain in them some fundamental element of our own selection and decision... it seems to have something to do with the value we place on autonomy, self-governance, self-authorship' (Mills, 1998, p.154). To determine whether it is in parents' interests to have genetic enhancement choices, I will now review existing theory on the value of having choices *per se*. Having choices is generally considered to contribute to a good life. However, it is difficult to articulate exactly what the value of choice *is*. In the literature, support has been given to both an instrumental and an intrinsic value of choice.

There are several ways in which having choices can be instrumentally valuable (Dworkin, 1988; Mills, 1998; Scanlon, 1988). First, having more than one option to choose from can increase potential well-being, as it may increase the probability people can obtain what they want. For example, parents would rather have a variety of schools to choose between, as this increases their chances of finding an environment they are satisfied with, and in which their child will flourish.

Second, the making of a choice may validate the existing options a person may have - a person would rather have chosen a particular outcome than be given it, even if a delegated outcome is what they would have wanted anyway. Suppose that our couple, Tom and Jane, have not yet been offered the choice I mentioned above. Suppose they are having difficulty conceiving a child and they begin to explore alternative options for having children, such as *In Vitro* Fertilisation, gamete donation and adoption. After evaluating the expense and risks involved in each alternative, they decide that they will not utilise any of these options. However, they say to their practitioner: 'We are glad that we at least now know that we will be childless by choice'. Tom and Jane are still in the same situation that they would have been in had they not been offered these options, but they believe their existing option has been validated by their decision not to utilise the alternatives.

A third instrumental value of choice is that the act of making a choice can allow scope for individuals to develop their character and gain self-knowledge. For example, if people were merely allocated to various relationships, vocations and lifestyles, they could be very happy with their situation, yet they would have missed out on the self-reflection and self-analysis that results from making these types of choices. Self-reflection is vital to our self-understanding, and if we are not able to make choices, then we may not gain valuable self-knowledge.

A final instrumental value of choice is that the act of making choices contributes to a person's role in society, as being allowed to make choices indicates social acceptance or belonging. For example, if a parent is judged by society to be unable to provide basic goods for their children, the State will usually intervene and remove the parents' right to care for the child or children affected. Here, the State has made a judgement that this parent is unable to fulfil their social role.

Although obviously important, these instrumental values do not, however, seem to capture what it is about choice that people fundamentally value. Does choice therefore have intrinsic value?

Numerous theorists have engaged in explanations of the factor that seems to be missing from the above descriptions of the instrumental value of choice. Claudia Mills suggests that above all else, the value of choice may be explained in the way that choices relate to living an *authentic* life (Mills, 1998, p.164). People want their lives to be something that they actively participate in and not merely something that happens to them. Further, choice can be considered as vital to a person's 'intentional agency', whereby a person expresses their agency better when they have choices, even if they are choosing what someone else would have given them anyway (Hurka, 1987, cited by Mills, 1998, p.158). Also relevant to both these values of choice are the kinds of choices a person has. If a person had a wide range of choices, but none of which were meaningful or all were awful, then this would not contribute to their authenticity as persons, or their 'intentional agency' (Mills, 1998, p.161).[4]

According to Dworkin however, choices do not have intrinsic value. He argues:

> Suppose someone ranks three goods A, B, and C in that order. Then… there will be A, B and C such that the person prefers a choice between B and C to receiving A. This will occur whenever the utility of having a choice between B and C plus the utility of B is greater than the utility of A. This seems to me irrational… why should I prefer to receive my second-ranked alternative to my first? (Dworkin, 1988, p.80)

However, Dworkin seems to overstate the significance of 'intrinsic value'. For even if choice does have intrinsic value, this does not imply that it has overriding value and should never be displaced. Anything of value always needs to be considered within the context of other things of value. Therefore, contrary to Dworkin's claim, I can value being given *A* more than I value choosing between *B* and *C* (the choice itself).

Yet suppose that Dworkin was correct, and having choices does not have intrinsic value. Does this matter? Perhaps not – as there is another value of choice that has yet to be discussed. According to Mills, what is valuable about choice is not the *exercise of choice* itself, but '... being recognised as the type of creature who is capable of making choices. That capacity grounds our idea of what it is to be a person and a moral agent equally worthy of respect by all' (Mills, 1998, p.161). Thus the value of choice is its contribution to people being recognised as agents capable of responsible decision-making. Having the ability to choose between options is generally better than simply having certain outcomes determined by another, as long as a meaningful range of choices is presented.

Avoiding problems with increased choice

I have suggested that choice is valuable as it contributes to people's moral agency and the authenticity of their actions. However, in examining this value of choice, I have given only minimal consideration to the optimum *amount* of choice that people should be presented with.

Several theorists have discussed the value of various 'amounts' of choice. For example, John Rawls included 'rights and liberties' in his list of primary goods (Rawls, 1971, p.92). He claimed that it is rational for any individual to be offered as much of any primary good as possible, as they 'are not compelled to accept more if they do not wish to' (Rawls, 1971, p.142-3). Thomas Hurka also stipulates that choices have a direct relationship with autonomy, whereby the ability to exercise more choice contributes to a freer life (Hurka, 1987).

However, extra choices are not costless. Gerald Dworkin, who argues that it can be rational not to increase choice, has provided the most detailed exploration of this problem (Dworkin, 1988). He relies upon several costs that having extra choices can engender. Three of these costs are considered here.[5]

First, factors such as the time involved in obtaining information about different options and the effort involved in making a decision between them ought to be recognised. Dworkin collects these under the heading of 'decision-making' or 'transaction' costs. This problem is also recognised by Harry Frankfurt, who in criticising Rawls' above position states:

> The assumption that it must always be better to have more of the primary goods rather than less implies that the marginal utility of an additional quantity of a primary good is invariably greater than its cost...[P]ossessing more of a primary good may well require

of a responsible individual that he spend more time and effort in managing it and in making decisions concerning its use. These activities are for many people intrinsically unappealing (Frankfurt, 1988, p.157).

Second, Dworkin has identified 'responsibility costs'. That is, responsibility arises when a person acts to bring about changes, as opposed to letting fate, chance or the decisions of others determine the future. As more choices become available, the moral responsibility of the person making the decision also accrues. People may not want increased moral responsibility when making choices.

Thirdly, a 'pressure to conform' also ought to be recognised. Even if there is more choice, the benefit of this could be undermined by social or legal sanctions that encourage individuals to make a particular choice. If this becomes the case, having more choices may not increase the actual number of choices at all.

When considering how much choice is desirable, these costs need to be evaluated. If a choice is introduced which does not meet these criteria, then it may merely add confusion, nuisance or inefficiency to the decision-making process. This may decrease the value of having this choice in the first place.

Is offering parents the choice of genetic enhancement good?

Parenthood signals a major upheaval in an individual's life. It alters social relationships, role demands and life structure (Salmela-Aro et al., 2000, p.171). The transition to parenthood involves several factors, including: planning to have a child, becoming pregnant and adapting to the pregnancy, childbirth and caring for the child. Vital to this process is an ability to make choices consistent with one's interests.

According to T. Schelling, the interests of parents may not be upheld if genetic enhancement choices were made available to them. He asks: '[w]ill people be glad to have this choice available? Or will it just add one more decision to make, one more source of conflict, one more opportunity for remorse, when life is already full enough of decisions?' (Schelling, 1978, p.200). Is there something about genetic enhancement choices that could create such problems? I will now utilise Dworkin's arguments above to identify three costs that parents may face in making these choices. Consider Tom and Jane again. In evaluating the option of enhancement via embryo selection, what processes would they have to undergo to consider the option? How responsible will they be for their decision to have a child via this process? What if they *feel* responsible? Would their choice truly be their own, or is there a potential for coercion? How harmful would this be?

Prior to addressing these questions, it is important to consider a preliminary but relevant issue. One of the most intuitively appealing reasons to explain the ethical significance of genetic research is that it allows for an ever-increasing role of deliberate intervention in human reproductive choices. An argument is often advanced that many genetic decisions should be 'left to chance', or that there is value in the 'genetic lottery'. Is it better to leave future development of genetic choices to chance? Ronald Dworkin thinks so. He argues that the 'crucial boundary between chance and choice is the spine of our ethics and our morality, and any serious shift in that boundary is seriously dislocating' (Dworkin, 1999). Here Dworkin is warning society not to proceed with unnecessary genetic interventions, as he is concerned that morality could be threatened if we deliberately allow things to become matters of choice, when they were previously left to chance alone. Thomas Schelling would support Dworkin's concern: '[t]here are some things… that it is a great relief to be unable to control. The lottery distributes arbitrary justice indiscriminately, but it may beat having to discriminate' (Schelling, 1978, p.203). Both Dworkin and Schelling would be concerned about being able to choose to distribute genetic choices for intelligence non-randomly.

However, whilst this concern is not trivial, the actuality of our current 'lack of control' in parental choice about intelligence is questionable, and there are several considerations that suggest that a person's genetic makeup is not determined entirely by chance. First, parents have been shown to 'assortatively' partner each other. That is, intelligent people tend to partner other intelligent people.[6] Additionally, parents seeking donor gametes for reproduction will often request information about the health and character of the gamete donor (Scheib, 1994). Thus although Dworkin and Schelling would presumably advocate the value of maintaining the 'genetic lottery', the actual behaviour of parents currently implies the opposite. Therefore, the value of chance alone cannot be a reason not to offer extra choices to parents.

Decision-making costs

What decision-making processes would Tom and Jane undergo to evaluate the option of enhancement via genetic selection? Could these be harmful? The choice to select for intelligence is not one that would be made frivolously by parents. To make an informed decision, parents would devote a significant amount of time and effort to examining the available options. They would also want to understand the technology involved, including any risks. Additionally, in selecting for intelligence, they would want to understand the personality, health and quality of life characteristics with which intelligence is correlated.

Further, decisions about genetic information are going to be more complex than those that parents currently face. Currently, most reproductive decisions that parents make will lead to an outcome where there is a high degree of certainty; for example whether or not a foetus carries known mutations of the gene involved with Cystic Fibrosis. In contrast, choices about traits of offspring will involve risks and trade-offs and will most likely not carry a guaranteed outcome. Consider the following scenario:

Researchers have recently announced that they have mapped over 125 genes contributing to human intelligence. Within these 125 genes, they identified at least 30 that they consider to be particularly important. However, a person did not need all 30 of these alleles to be 'intelligent', a selection of 12 – 17 of them was considered to be enough to contribute to an above-average intelligence score. The authors also claimed that there might be other significant genes that had not been mapped yet. Parents who want to select for intelligence are to be presented with a table of probability, which correlates the presence of different numbers and types of 'intelligence' genes with an ability test score range.

This scenario is a simplistic representation of the kind of information genetic research into intelligence could provide. However, it illustrates the complexity that beginning to utilise this information in reproductive decision-making could lead to.

An important aspect of considering decision-making costs is evaluating how parents will comprehend and respond to complex behavioural genetic information. To date, there has been virtually no empirical research undertaken to examine people's knowledge and attitudes towards behavioural genetic information.[7] However, many studies have been undertaken which gauge understanding of genetic information about complex genetic diseases. Evidence from these studies suggests that due recognition is given to both genetic and environmental contributions to multifactorial traits (Richards, 1997; Richards, 1996).

One study however is particularly interesting. A pilot study by Senior et al. (1999) examined parents' perceptions of health information about their infant children, in the context of familial hypercholesterolemia. This disease has a genetic predisposition, but is controllable by diet and drug therapy. Here, the researchers provided the information about hypercholestrolemia to parents phrased as either diagnostic information, or as the results of a genetic test. They found that when the test was seen as detecting a genetic problem, the condition was perceived as uncontrollable and, hence, more threatening. Two mothers in the study stated that: '[i]t's the word hereditary that sets the alarm bells ringing… it sort of suggests that there is nothing you can do about it. Hereditary levels, as I understand it, cannot be affected by diet. So you know, I feel as though this death sentence has been put on my little boy' (Senior, et al., 1999, p.1859). This finding is interesting, as it indicates that although there may be good 'population-based' knowledge about the causes of complex genetic disease, once that information is applied on an individual level, this can then lead to a greater emphasis upon genetic information, discounting of other relevant factors. This could also have implications for the children of these parents who were provided with genetic information, as this could affect parents' subsequent behaviour in minimising the potential for disease.

This choice of genetic selection for intelligence is at risk of creating a serious decision-making cost. If these attitudes of individuals and parents towards genetic information remain consistent across the spectrum of genetic traits, then parents such as Tom and Jane may adopt a determinist attitude when considering the development of intelligence. Their choice, combined with their potentially fatalistic attitude towards behavioural genetic information, could mean that they are constantly 'watching and waiting' for their child's intelligence to develop, and this could have implications for how they develop a relationship with their child.

However, it should also be recognised that this potential for over-emphasising genetic information will not necessarily harm the interests of *all* parents who are considering genetic enhancement. Just as there will be parents who may over-interpret the significance of genetic involvement in the development of intelligence, it is reasonable to assume that not all parents will be fatalistic. Parents' attitudes to probabilistic information are likely to be context-sensitive; dependent upon the attitudes they have about both the nature of intelligence and their knowledge of genetics, their personal goals, the other options they have available, and the consequences of choosing as opposed to not choosing a particular intelligence profile (Lappé, 1993, p.58). Further, Scarr has shown that once people become aware of their own talents or shortcomings, they take an active role to try and shape their environment accordingly (Cited by Terwogt, et al., 1993, p.499). It is reasonable to assume that parents would adopt a similar role with their selected children.

Increased, unwanted responsibility?

Another cost of having extra choices is that choosing among a greater number of choices may also create a higher level of responsibility for the choice made. According to Strong: '[w]hen offspring characteristics are under parental control... there would be a greater tendency to blame parents for their children's imperfections. The question, "Can't you control your children?" might take on a darker meaning' (Strong, 2001, p.13). Should parents be held more morally accountable for the outcome of a pregnancy if the pregnancy was established via genetic selection than if the child had been conceived naturally? Is this something that parents are going to want? If parents make a deliberate choice, then arguably they could be held accountable for the outcome. Consider Tom and Jane again. Say that they decided to choose the potential intelligence of their child. At age 10, their child is very bright, but has an anxiety disorder. Would Jane be justified in feeling responsible for her child's anxiety?

Here, Jane's responsibility may be contingent upon the information that they had at the time of making their choice. If there was a known association between higher intelligence and anxiety, then they could be held responsible for this outcome. If they did not know of this risk, or the risk was not significant, then they are no more responsible for their child's anxiety than is any other parent.

Yet even if Tom and Jane did have information about anxiety at the time of choosing their embryo, this should not automatically render them responsible. If Tom and Jane in good faith believed that in choosing an embryo with higher potential intelligence, this would give the resulting child the best possible life, then it is not clear that they are morally responsible for a sub-optimal outcome.

However, say there is some greater responsibility in making a deliberate choice in procreation. Is this something that Tom and Jane are going to want to accept? Here, the implications of deliberate choices can be evaluated by examining empirical outcomes where parents have made such a choice in procreation.

An excellent example of a deliberate choice in procreation is that of existing couples who have chosen assisted reproductive technology in order to have children. Of this, the case that best mirrors the problem under examination here is that of parents who undergo in-vitro fertilisation with their own gametes. Are parents of IVF children more harmed by the responsibility they have for their procreative decisions than parents who have not utilised IVF?

Many empirical studies have been undertaken in following up over 20 years of parental decisions to utilise IVF technology. Although these studies have not directly assessed whether parents feel harmed by their responsibility, they have examined factors that are reflective of responsibility, including emotional involvement, separation anxiety, perceptions of vulnerability and parental expectations of children.

The majority of these longitudinal studies have indicated that parents who have conceived children utilising IVF technology are not worse-off (and may be better-off) than those who have conceived children using other means (See, eg: Braverman et al., 1998; Golombok et al., 1995; Golombok et al., 2001; McMahon et al., 1997; Weaver et al., 1993). They generally found no differences between IVF parents and parents who had conceived naturally with respect to adjustment to parenthood, or the burden they feel in being parents. These studies have also indicated that parents of IVF children did not place excessive expectations for achievement upon their children, that they were more emotionally involved with their child, and that they were not over-protective or worried about their child.

However, some of these studies have also indicated that IVF mothers saw their children as more vulnerable, and that they can exhibit separation anxiety when compared to non-IVF mothers (Colpin et al, 1995; Hahn and DiPietro, 2001). This could indicate that IVF parents may exhibit an increased sense of responsibility for their children. However, authors have suggested that appropriate counselling could mitigate this potential problem and these differences have all but disappeared in parents of teenaged IVF children (Golombok et al., 2001). These studies therefore suggest that if there is an increase in parental responsibility through enhancement choices, that parents are not routinely going to be harmed as a result.

Pressure to make a particular choice

Perhaps the most serious potential cost to parents of choosing the intelligence of their children is that, when faced with the availability of genetic enhancement, parents will feel compelled to use this technology, regardless of their personal attitudes or values. Consider Tom and Jane again:

> Tom and Jane have decided to proceed with in-vitro fertilisation in order to try and have a child. At one of their consultations, the doctor advises them that it is also possible to selectively implant embryos, and that intelligence is a trait that they can predict with some confidence. He offers them counselling so that they can discuss this option, and off-handedly remarks that more and more parents are now choosing this additional procedure. In the car on the way home, Tom remarks to Jane: 'Well, if everyone else is doing it, we better do it too. After all, intelligence is good, isn't it?'.

This vignette raises numerous questions. First, is there a potential for coercion to effectively force parents to make a particular decision? Second, if the factor directing parents is not coercive, what is it? Third, even if there is a potential for influence in parents decisions, is this 'acceptable'?

Coercion is broadly construed as the presence of unreasonable external pressures or constraints one faces when making a decision. According to Beauchamp and Childress: '[c]oercion ... occurs if and only if one person intentionally uses a credible and severe threat of harm or force to control another' (Beauchamp and Childress, 1994, p.164). Thus coercion exists when there is effectively no choice but to perform a particular act, even if theoretically a person has more than one choice. A coercive threat is made intentionally, and it involves threatening harm to those who do not bow to the coercer's will. As Schelling points out, it is not difficult to imagine such influences upon parents' decisions to utilise genetic selection for intelligence: 'if it became widely believed in social classes that nearly everybody was taking advantage of this opportunity; parents might feel coerced into practising selection not out of any dissatisfaction with the prospective intelligence of their children, but to keep up with the new generation' (Schelling, 1978, p.208). On the above definition of coercion however, it is not obvious that Tom and Jane are facing a *coercive* threat. What they are experiencing is more an awareness of their current social environment; looking to the decisions that other couples are making, and utilising those in making their own decision. There has not been an unreasonable threat made directly towards them, and it is not clear that they will suffer harm if they do not choose genetic enhancement. This offer may involve pressure to conform, but it is not harmful to Tom and Jane in the way that most coercive offers are.

However although Tom and Jane are not necessarily being subjected to coercion, some may argue that there may still be elements of the selection decision process that may be harmful to Tom and Jane's interests in procreative autonomy. I term these elements the 'dominant social interests' influencing reproductive decisions. Numerous ethicists have already commented on these. According to Agar: 'popular suggestions such as the avoidance of disease or the securing of quality of life threaten to smuggle into individual choices substantive views about human worth... citizens will end up being engineered in accordance with a dominant set of values' (Agar, 1998, p.137). This may extend to non-medical traits. A recent study indicates that, whilst still small, public support for selecting desirable traits in children is increasing (Marteau et al., 1995). Evidence for expectations on parents to utilise screening for diseases such as Down's syndrome is well-documented (See, eg: Gekas et al., 1999; Marteau and Drake, 1995; Smith, et al., 1994; Tymstra, 1989). Additionally, Michie and Marteau claim that parents evaluate their options based on social meanings and social consequences, and not on biomedical risk information or abstract ethical principles (Michie and Marteau, 1996, p.110). Thus the influence of 'dominant social interests', although less sinister than coercion, may hold a significant potential for adversely impacting upon the choices that parents make.

However, in criticising the 'dominant social values' that permeate our ability to make truly informed decisions, are we attempting to question something that is simply impossible to avoid? After all, we live in a society where many of the decisions we make are influenced by factors from our environment, advertising being a good example. To argue against dominant social interests influencing genetic enhancement choices may be to fail to recognise that some element of influence may be intricately and inextricably entwined with the availability of this new technology.

Obviously parents will have feelings of connectivity and responsibility to their future child, which will affect their decision.[8] We should recognise that: 'moral and emotional commitments are not exceptional, are not constraints on freedom, but are rather a part of ordinary human life' (Crouch and Elliott, 1999, p.278). To perceive an element of influence in wanting the best for your child may therefore simply indicate that one is a caring parent, with moral and emotional commitments to one's child. The challenge is to ensure that these external influences are legitimate. As Mills states:

> [W]e will always be making our choices against the background of others' predicted or actual reactions to those choices, so we cannot expect to make our choices in a moral vacuum, influenced by nothing. Others can legitimately seek to influence us in our choices; we distinguish between legitimate and illegitimate influence according to the means used...(Mills, 1998, p.161).

Conclusion

The consequences of making genetic enhancement choices are significant and potentially costly. Through an analysis of the value of having and increasing the choices that people can make, I have identified and evaluated the potential harms that genetic enhancement choices could have for parents.

I have argued that the choice of genetic enhancement may carry some costs, but that it is unlikely these will offer overwhelming risks to parents. However, this does not mean that genetic enhancement will always be in parents' best interests, and it is certainly not a decision that all parents are going to want to make. If any parents do decide to make such a choice, it is vital that they are made fully aware of the potential harms of genetic selection choices in order to give fully informed consent.

Additionally, we should recognise that there will be great diversity in parents' attitudes towards this technology and that individual values and experiences will be important. Parents will make decisions based upon their perception of harm, the value they place on the trait, their personal experiences and the attitudes of others. Thus the most sensible action will be to *proceed slowly.*

Notes

1 This chapter has benefited from discussions held with Julian Savulescu, David McCarthy and Lynn Gillam. Additionally, the author thanks for their commentary the staff at the Centre for the Study of Health and Society, The University of Melbourne, and delegates at the Society for Applied Philosophy Annual Conference 2000.

2 This could be achieved in one of two ways: genetic selection (where embryos with a particular genetic predisposition are selectively implanted during in-vitro fertilisation) or genetic engineering (where the DNA of an embryo is altered).

3 Objections to genetic enhancement include claims that it will harm the future autonomy of the individual born, lead to an overly competitive society, create greater social inequity and be a bad allocation of medical resources. Specific responses to the various objections can include claims that persons are not 'directed' by their genetic material, that these interventions are not significantly different from current parental interventions, and that the real challenge actually lies in protecting people from overbearing parents, regardless of genetic information or genetic intervention. Therefore, for the purposes of this chapter, it will be assumed that these objections are not substantial, and that genetic enhancement is either neutral or beneficial for the person being born (See, eg: Caplan et al., 1999, Glover, 1984, Harris, 1998b).

4 Here she cites Raz's examples of the 'man in the pit' and the 'hounded woman', both of whom have a large number of choices but do not lead autonomous, free lives (Raz, 1986).

5 It is important to note that Dworkin deliberately does not consider one cost: 'If A says to B that if B offered more options with respect to some matter, A will kill B.' Dworkin points out that in rejecting A's offer, B rejects the additional choices not because of the nature of the choices, nor the choosing per se, but the arbitrary cost attached to the increase in choice.

6 This is consistent with the requirement (discussed above) that additional options be meaningful, and that they do not directly cause harm.

7 'Assortative mating' refers to the tendency of people to select a partner according to particular characteristics they have, such as physical characteristics. The correlation between partners for IQ is approximately 0.33–0.40. This correlation grows to 0.60 when the factor is education. (See, eg: Bouchard and McGue, 1981, Jensen, 1978.)

8 Personal Communication, Professor Theresa Marteau, August 10, 2000. A reason for this gap in research could be because the experts themselves do not know what the predictive significance of this information will be.

9   A parallel example here is that of living organ donation between family members (See, eg: Crouch and Elliott, 1999). Here coercion has been raised as one reason why perhaps family members should not be offered the choice of saving another family member – another family member may find it too hard to say 'no' to donating a compatible organ because of their feelings of altruism towards another member of their family.

References

Agar, N. (1998), 'Liberal eugenics', *Public affairs quarterly,* vol. 12(2), pp.137-155.

Beauchamp, T.L., and Childress, J.F. (1994), *Principles of biomedical ethics,* 4th ed, Oxford, Oxford University Press.

Bouchard, T.J. Jr. and McGue, M. (1981), 'Familial studies of intelligence: a review', *Science,* vol. 212, pp.1055-1059.

Braverman, A.M., Boxer, A.S., Corson, S.L., Coutifaris, C. and Hendrix, A. (1998), 'Characteristics and attitudes of parents of children born with the use of assisted reproductive technology', *Fertility and Sterility,* vol. 70(5), pp.860-865.

Caplan, A.L., McGee, G. and Magnus, D. (1999), 'What is immoral about eugenics?', *BMJ,* vol. 319, pp.1284-1285.

Colpin, H., Demyttenaere, K. and Vandemeulebroecke, L. (1995), 'New reproductive technology and the family: The parent-child relationship following *in vitro* fertilization', *Journal of Child Psychology and Psychiatry,* vol. 36(8), pp.1429-1441.

Crouch, R.A. and Elliott, C. (1999), 'Moral agency and the family: the case of living-related organ transplantation', *Cambridge Quarterly of Healthcare Ethics,* vol. 8, pp.275-287.

Dworkin, G. (1988), 'Is More Choice Better than Less?', in (his) *The Theory and Practice of Autonomy,* Cambridge, Cambridge University Press, pp.62-81.

Dworkin, R. (1999), 'Justice and fate: an introductory paper to genetics, identity and justice', available at: http://www.21stcenturytrust.org/genetics.doc (accessed August 12, 2001).

Frankfurt, H. (1988), 'Equality as a moral ideal', in (his) *The Importance Of What We Care About: Philosophical Essays,* Cambridge and New York, Cambridge University Press, pp.134-158.

Gekas, J., Gondry, J., Mazur, S., Cesbron, S., Cesbron, P. and Thepot, F. (1999), 'Informed consent to serum screening for Down syndrome: Are women given adequate information?', *Prenatal Diagnosis,* vol. 19, pp.1-7.

Glover, J. (1984), *What Sort Of People Should There Be?,* Hammondsworth, Penguin.

Golombok, S., Cook, R., Bish, A. and Murray, C. (1995), 'Families created by the new reproductive technologies: Quality of parenting and social and emotional development of children', *Child Development,* vol. 66, pp.285-298.

Golombok, S., MacCallum, F. and Goodman, E. (2001), 'The 'test-tube' generation: parent-child relationships and the psychological well-being of in vitro fertilization children at adolescence', *Child Development,* vol. 72(2), pp.599-608.

Hahn, C.S. and DiPietro, J.A. (2001), 'In vitro fertilisation and the family: Quality of parenting, family functioning, and child psychosocial adjustment', *Developmental Psychology,* vol. 37(1), pp.37-48.

Harris, J. (1997), ''Goodbye Dolly?' The ethics of human cloning', *Journal of Medical Ethics,* vol. 23, pp.353-360.

Harris, J. (1998a), 'Rights and Reproductive Choice', in Harris, J. and Holm, S. (eds), *The Future of Human Reproduction*, Oxford, Clarendon Press, pp.5-37.

Harris, J. (1998b), *Clones, Genes and Immortality*, Oxford, Oxford University Press.

Hurka, T. (1987), 'Why value autonomy?', *Social Theory and Practice*, vol. 13, pp.361-82.

Jensen, A. (1978) 'Genetic and behavioral effects of nonrandom mating', in Osborne, R.T.O., Noble, C.E. and Weyl, N. (eds), *Human variation: The biopsychology of age, race, and sex*, New York, Academic Press, pp.51-105.

Lappé, M. (1993), 'Risk and the ethics of genetic choice, in Bartels, D.M. LeRoy, B.S. and Caplan, A.L. (eds), *Prescribing our future: ethical challenges in genetic counselling*, New York, Aldine De Gruyter, pp.57-63.

Marteau, T.M. and Drake, H. (1995), 'Attributions for disability: the influence of genetic screening', *Social Science and Medicine*, vol. 40(8), pp.1127-1132.

Marteau, T., Michie, S., Drake, H. and Bobrow, M. (1995), 'Public attitudes towards the selection of desirable characteristics in children', *Journal of Medical Genetics*, vol. 32, pp.796-798.

McMahon, C.A., Ungerer, J.A., Tennant, C. and Saunders, D. (1997), 'Psychological adjustment and the quality of the mother-child relationship at four months postpartum after conception by in vitro fertilization', *Fertility and Sterility*, vol. 68(3), pp.492-500.

Michie, S. and Marteau, T. (1996), 'Genetic counselling: some issues of theory and practice', in Marteau, T. and Richards, M. (eds), *The troubled helix: social and psychological implications of the new human genetics*, Cambridge, Cambridge University Press, pp.104-122.

Mills, C. (1998), 'Choice and Circumstance', *Ethics*, vol. 109, pp.154-165.

Parfit, D. (1984), *Reasons and Persons,* Oxford, Oxford University Press.

Rawls, J. (1971), *A Theory Of Justice*, Oxford, Oxford University Press.

Raz, J. (1986), *The Morality of Freedom*, Oxford, Oxford University Press.

Richards, M. (1996), 'Lay and professional knowledge of genetics and inheritance', *Public Understanding of Science*, vol. 5, pp.217-230.

Richards, M. (1997), 'It runs in the family: lay knowledge about genetic inheritance', in Clarke, A. and Parsons, E. (eds), *Culture, Kinship and Genes: towards cross-cultural genetics*, Basingstoke, Macmillan Press, pp.175-194.

Robertson, J.A. (1994), *Children Of Choice: Freedom And The New Reproductive Technologies*, Princeton, NJ, Princeton University Press.

Salmela-Aro, K., Nurmi, J. E., Saisto, T. and Halmesmaki, E. (2000), 'Women's and men's personal goals during the transition to parenthood', *Journal of Family Psychology*, vol. 14(2), pp.171-86.

Scanlon, T. (1988), 'The significance of choice: Lecture 2, The Value of Choice', *The Tanner Lectures on Human Values*, vol. 8, pp.177-185.

Scheib, J. (1994), 'Sperm donor selection and the psychology of female mate choice', *Ethology and Sociobiology*, vol. 15, pp.113-129.

Schelling, T. (1978), 'Choosing our children's genes', in (his) *Micromotives and Macrobehaviour*, New York, Norton, pp.193-210.

Senior, V., Marteau, T.M. and Peters, T.J. (1999), 'Will genetic testing for predisposition for disease result in fatalism? A qualitative study of parents responses to neonatal screening for familial hypercholesterolaemia', *Social Science and Medicine*, vol. 48(12), pp.1857-60.

Smith, D.K., Shaw, R.W. and Marteau, T.M. (1994), 'Informed consent to undergo serum screening for Down's syndrome: the gap between policy and practice', *BMJ*, vol. 309, pp.776.

Strong, C. (2001), ' Can't you control your children?', *American Journal of Bioethics*, vol. 1(1), pp.12-13.

Terwogt, M.M., Hoeksma, J.B. and Koops, W. (1993), 'Common beliefs about the heredity of human characteristics', *British journal of psychology*, vol. 84(4), pp.499-503.

Tymstra, T. (1989) 'The imperative character of medical technology and the meaning of 'anticipated decision regret', *International Journal of Technology Assessment in Health Care*, vol. 5, pp.207-213.

Weaver, S.M., Clifford, E., Gordon, A.G., Hay, D.M. and Robinson, J. (1993), 'A follow-up study of 'successful' IVF/GIFT couples: social-emotional well-being and adjustment to parenthood', *Journal of Psychosomatic Obstetrics & Gynaecology*, vol. 14(Suppl), pp.5-16.

Chapter 4

The Child's Right to an Open Future and Modern Genetics[1]

Tuija Takala

The previous chapter has focused on the question of whether to make use of the new possibilities of genetic choice at the embryonic stage from the point of view of the parents. In this chapter, I consider the issue from the perspective of the possible resulting child. I do this by focusing on an important argument put forward by the philosopher Joel Feinberg in favour of a child's right to an open future. I ask, is there such a right, and, if so, does it preclude a parental decision to make use of the PGD (preimplantation genetic diagnosis)? Let me begin with an imaginary picture:

> A wealthy professional couple with two healthy children. The family lives in a beautiful country house with a garden and a swimming pool, not too far from the nearby city. Their lives are joyful and laughter often echoes in the premises. Parents seldom leave the house, computers allow them to work at home. The children spend their days playing in the garden. Everyone is happy. The children are 12 and 14 years of age. They have never been to school and do not know how to read, write or count.

Why do we think that there is something wrong with this picture? Why is it wrong that 12 and 14 year-olds cannot read or write? Why is school so important? The children are happy – is that not the main thing? One response to this is that we are concerned for the *future* of the children – in fact, more concerned for their future than for their happiness *now*. Joel Feinberg has given this a philosophical formulation in his paper 'the child's right to an open future' (Feinberg, 1992, pp.76-97).

The 'child's right to an open future' argument centres on the protection of autonomy, that is, on the child's right *not* to have her future options irrevocably foreclosed. The argument has been used in applied ethics to analyse which of the decisions made by parents and other adults on behalf of minors are justifiable and which are not. The classical cases are the refusal of life-saving treatment and the denial of basic education (Feinberg, 1992, pp.76-97). Problems arise in these cases when the moral, political or religious convictions of the parents conflict with what is considered by others to be in the best interests of the child, in terms of her future autonomy. The traditional open-future arguments concern *infants* and *children*, but they are applicable to *fetuses* as well. This extension has apparently suggested that the model can also be used to solve some of the ethical problems created by modern genetics – particularly by *preimplantation genetic diagnosis* (PGD) and *fetal gene therapy*. The justification of these is, after all (at least partly) the good of the 'future child'. But tempting as the idea may be, the fact that it is in these cases ultimately unclear who 'the child' is creates problems. And furthermore, Feinberg's theory on the right to an open future, when brought to bear on genetics, can be interpreted in different, even contradictory, ways. In this chapter I will analyse whether the open-future argument is applicable to the ethical problems of modern genetics at all and even if it is, whether it helps to solve those problems.

The classical cases and a new one

An oft-quoted case in biomedical ethics is the refusal of Jehovah's Witnesses to accept even life-saving blood transfusions.[2] When a minor is in question, the open-future argument seems easily applicable. If the child dies, her future autonomy is, among other things, restricted most severely, since it no longer exists. And in most countries it is the doctors' duty to save the child in these cases regardless of her parents' wishes.

Joel Feinberg uses the even more controversial example of Amish communities and the struggle of Amish parents to keep their children away from state-accredited schools. The Amish live in simple self-sufficient farming communities along religious principles. They wish to keep the secular and technological influences of modern societies excluded from their traditional lifestyle. In their view, sending their children to public schools would undermine the very foundations of their tradition. According to Feinberg, the open-future argument entails that Amish children should, regardless of their parents' wishes, have the same minimal education as every other child. If we fail to give them this, their future options will not include careers outside the Amish community.[3] On the other hand, should the children attend a 'normal' school until the age of sixteen, it might be difficult for them to go back to Amish life. In this sense, it is not only the Amish culture that is at stake but also the child's future right to remain a part of her own original culture.

Dena S. Davis has used the open-future argument in yet another context in her paper 'Genetic Dilemmas and the Child's Right to an Open Future' (1997, pp.7-15). The ethical problems she deals with are brought about by *in vitro fertilisation* and *preimplantation genetic diagnosis* – methods by which parents can, to a certain degree, select their offspring.[4] The specific dilemma Davis focuses on in her paper is the issue of deaf parents who wish to have a deaf child.

With the modern gene technologies hereditary deafness can be avoided. It is possible to select embryos with non-defective genes for implantation and this method can be used to avoid the birth of a deaf child in the first place. According to an oft-used justification for doing this, deafness is a disability and disabilities should be avoided. But because the claim that deafness is a disability can be, and has been, challenged, Davis concedes with the deaf activists, that deafness can also be seen as a separate culture. In her reading of the open-future argument even this would, however, lead us to conclude that deafness, when avoidable, should be avoided:

> If deafness is considered a disability, one that substantially narrows a child's career, marriage, and cultural options in the future, then deliberately creating a deaf child counts as a moral harm. If deafness is considered a culture, as Deaf activists would have us agree, then deliberately creating a deaf child who will have only very limited options to move outside of that culture, also counts as moral harm (Davis, 1997, p.14).

On the surface it seems that she is following Feinberg's argument. Further analysis shows, however, that this is not necessarily the case.

Epistemic versus moral arrogance

Those who defend the rights of the children against the cultural claims of their parents are often accused of arrogance and 'moral imperialism'. Sometimes these accusations are justifiable, but cases differ.

Feinberg's argument in the case of Amish children is, at the most, epistemically arrogant. If the world continues to be what it is and to 'develop' in ways we can foresee – the economic structures, the institutions, the states, the professions and the like will stay basically the same and there will be no global catastrophe that forces the survivors to start again from scratch – as Feinberg seems to believe, then it is plausible to argue that children will be better off, in terms of their future options and autonomy, if they go to school for the required years.

Davis's argument, on the other hand, seems to be more open to accusations of moral arrogance. If deafness is considered a disability that substantially narrows the child's future options, then the open-future argument can perhaps be applied. But if deafness is not considered a disability but a culture from which it is difficult to part, then the suitability of the open-future argument is not clear. As a blue-eyed and fair-haired person I assume that I would have considerable obstacles should I choose to join the Black culture. As a woman I cannot really be one of the lads, and as a city person I would have difficulties trying to assimilate to agrarian communities. Had someone deliberately created me this way, would she have violated my right to an open future? I do not think so. All people are born, and belong, to various communities.

There is a significant difference in the cases presented by Feinberg and Davis. Feinberg does not say that there is something wrong or less valuable about Amish communities *per se*. He only notes that many career options and life style choices are not available to the Amish *children* if they are deprived of normal schooling. Therefore, in the name of their open future, they should have the same basic education as the rest. Davis, on the other hand, seems to argue that belonging to the deaf culture is in itself a harm, because it forecloses the children the option to leave that culture. But this argument presupposes a value judgement regarding the deaf community. We cannot say that an individual's future options are limited simply because she belongs to one culture rather than to another (as everyone belongs to some culture[s] in any case), unless we are also prepared to say that some cultures are better or worse than others.

When does the right to an open future begin?

Within the past few decades the moral problems we face in terms of the good of our offspring have changed. In her paper, Davis extends the application of the open-future argument to a new sphere. The examples Feinberg gives deal with existing individuals. Davis, in her turn, is talking about possible future human beings. What would it mean to talk about the child's right to an open future in relation to, say, six embryos *in vitro*, out of whom only two will be given the chance to live? If they all have a right to an open future, we should withdraw from using IVF ever again. It would be dangerous to implant all six, and it would be wrong to give only one or two of them the chance to live. In either case we would violate someone's right to an open future. If, on the other hand, the embryos only have a *potential* right to an open future, due to the possibility that they might someday become persons whose future option should be kept open, the open-future argument would not, as such, apply to them.

When we choose the embryos for implantation, the open-future argument does not oblige us to choose the fittest of them. There is (as far as we know) no pre-chosen 'child' just waiting to be assigned a genetic composition by medical professionals, ethics committees, by her parents or by nature. Under favourable conditions all six embryos would develop into separate persons. It can be decided that the embryo with genetic defects is not implanted, while the embryo with no known defects is. But this cannot be justified by an appeal to the 'child's right to an open future', as there is no *one* possible future child to begin with, but *two* embryos with different genetic makeups who would, given the opportunity, develop into two different children. In order to employ the open-future argument, it is necessary to postulate a pre-person for whom the future options are kept open. Therefore, the open-future argument *cannot* justify our choice of one embryo over another for implantation.

I shall disregard all the questions concerning abortion here (is it justifiable, on what conditions and during which trimester, to mention but a few) and work on the presumption that if it is decided that a certain embryo or fetus will be carried to term so that it can, in the future, become a person, then it does have a right to an open future. Within this view, those embryos and fetuses which are intended to be born can be said to have the right to an open future. Let us now consider cases where the open-future argument might apply but is yet challenged by the possibilities created by modern genetics.

Genes and the open future

In Feinberg's open-future essay the tone of his argument is difficult to interpret as other than reductionist (or biologist). He is well aware that every decision regarding the upbringing and education of one's offspring will limit their future options, and thus, that no child's future can be kept entirely open (Feinberg, 1992, p.93). To resolve this potential paradox he asks us to consider infants:

> Right from the beginning the newborn infant has a kind of rudimentary character consisting of temperamental proclivities and *genetically fixed potential* for the acquisition of various talents and skills (Feinberg, 1992, p.95, italics added).

According to Feinberg, it is in relation to these 'natural' tendencies that the future options of the child should be kept open. And this is what the right to an open future means in practice. We should work to promote the satisfaction of the child's natural preferences, to strengthen her basic tendencies, and to keep her growth 'natural' (Feinberg, 1992, p.97). The person whose future autonomy should be protected is the biological entity, with her particular set of (inherited) genes, and her open future is to be measured in relation to what her genes have preconditioned her to become.

If our genetic constitution profoundly determines the person we are, it seems impossible to use Feinberg's open-future argument, as such, to justify the use of gene therapy of any kind. Although one could, of course, argue that *once* genetic modifications *have been made* (for whatever reasons, justified or unjustified), then the open-future argument becomes useful again. In this case it would just be a *different* genetic composition against which the question 'What is best for this child in terms of her future autonomy?' should be tested. This, however, is not an application of the open-future argument to solve the ethical problems of modern genetics but a mere reaction to the altered situation after gene therapy has already been performed. On the other hand, it could, I suppose, be argued that the 'natural growth' of a child is not determined by her genes alone, but that there is a soul (or some other spiritual entity) which, for its part, shapes her natural tendencies. There is, however, no evidence in Feinberg's essay that he would have meant this.

One possible route to save the open-future argument would be to assert that being 'healthy' is somehow a precondition for 'natural' growth. This would mean that genetic mutations that cause 'diseases' are in and by themselves obstacles to the natural growth of a person and should therefore be, in the name of the 'right to an open future' removed.[5] In the context of Davis's article, this only begs the question, as her point is to say that (deliberately chosen) deafness violates the child's right to an open future even if deafness is *not* considered to be a disability or a disease. She employs the open-future argument precisely because there is no consensus on whether deafness is a disability or not. But let us assume, for argument's sake (and because it is done so often in this discussion), that it is somehow easy to separate the disabled from the non-disabled and that there are no moral problems in discriminating against the disabled (by not letting them be born).[6]

Genetic enhancements and the open future

If it is assumed that disabilities, in this case those caused by genetic defects, are obstacles to the child's natural growth and to her open future, what would follow from Feinberg's open-future considerations? Severe defects will, without a doubt, limit the future child's options in life (as compared to those of a healthy child), and thus, when such defects can be avoided, the necessary medical procedures should be carried out in an early stage. And minor deviations from the norm, too, will limit the future person's options. A child with a hereditary less-than-average IQ will have restricted career opportunities, and an individual with physical abnormalities will experience more problems in her social life than her healthy peers. The child's right to an open future, however, seems to demand us to go even further.

What is interesting in Feinberg's Amish-children example is that it presents a 'natural' situation where affirmative action is needed to enhance and to secure the child's future autonomy. With genetic defects we have been talking about removing obstacles, but with the Amish children the question seems to be one of creating opportunities that would not have been there 'naturally'. Similar demands should perhaps be applied to others as well. At conception the fetuses have 'received' their 'natural' genes, just as the Amish children have become part of their 'natural' culture by birth. Why are we morally required to improve the situation of the latter but not the former? If 'the right to an open future' is taken seriously (with the given presupposition) we ought to conclude that we should, when it becomes possible, genetically enhance our future offspring to meet at least the average human level of functioning. This is what the child's right to an open future demands us to do in terms of future opportunities created by schooling: the child to have at least the same opportunities as all the other children have.

Of course Feinberg did not, and probably would not, say this. To reach this conclusion I replaced Feinberg's reductionist view with an even more restricted view, according to which a person is profoundly her genes, minus defects. Nevertheless, something that goes beyond Feinberg's definitions is needed if one wishes to use Feinberg's open-future argument to deal with the ethical problems arising from modern genetics.

Are we our genes?

Feinberg's argument from the open future claims, among other things, that in protecting the child's future autonomy we should consider her 'natural' talents and features as indicators of what her autonomous self, when it emerges, will want. Maybe this is simply the best we can do and not a strong statement on what people fundamentally are. If we want to protect a child's future autonomy, we should look for the signs of 'what the child is likely to want in the future' from the child herself and not elsewhere. Her 'natural' features are the most likely candidate for a source of impartial information.

It is difficult to see how the open-future argument could solve any of the ethical problems created by modern genetics. It is applicable only after a 'pre-person' exists. In the sense that Feinberg uses the 'right to an open future' it means that we should keep *that child's own* future options open in view of *natural features*. It cannot say whether these or those natural features are better than others. These are questions which need to be tackled with other concepts, such as 'the right to life', 'the right to avoid suffering', 'the right to reproduce' and so forth.

If we, nevertheless, try to use the open-future argument (with modifications) to the ethical problems of genetics, we can come either to the conclusion that no genetic modifications are to be condoned or to the conclusion that every child should be enhanced to meet at least the average human condition. These are both plausible conclusions, depending on the premises chosen. There are, of course, other possibilities, depending on the modifications made to the original argument.

When applied in the sphere of ethical dilemmas created by genetics, the open-future argument revealed some of its weaknesses. The strong commitment to the 'natural, genetically fixed potential' as the indicator of who we are, is a controversial metaphysical presupposition, even if practical and sometimes intuitive. Moreover, the epistemic arrogance that the open-future argument displays is not completely unproblematic, as it demands us to take Feinberg's beliefs about the future of the world as material conditions for what a child's right to an open future should include.

When it comes to the traditional questions of biomedical ethics, Feinberg's open-future argument is clearly not without merit. As a liberal answer to the question, 'how should we treat minors', it has well proven its place. As such, it cannot, however, answer the ethical questions brought to the fore by modern genetics. Feinberg's paper clarifies insufficiently just those concepts and presuppositions which would be crucial tools for us to be able to tackle the new questions.

Notes

1   My thanks are due to Simo Vehmas, University of Jyväskylä, Finland.

2   See e.g. Harris, J. (1985), *The Value of Life*. London, Routledge & Kegan Paul, pp.202-3 and 216; H. Tristram Engelhardt, Jr. (1996), *The Foundations of Bioethics* [2nd ed.], Oxford, Oxford University Press, pp.329-330; T.L. Beauchamp and J.F. Childress (1983), *Principles of Biomedical Ethics*, Oxford, Oxford University Press, p.138.

3   Feinberg (1992), pp.81-97. His example is based on the court cases *State v. Garber* (1966) and *Wisconsin v. Yoder, et al.* (1972) and has been simplified here.

4   On the matter of how much it is the parents' choice and related problems, see, e.g., H. Draper, and R. Chadwick (1999), 'Beware! Preimplantation genetic diagnosis may solve some old problems but it also raises new ones', *Journal of Medical Ethics* vol. 25, pp.114-120.

5   The view that diseases are not part of a 'natural' person has been endorsed e.g. by the German Enquete commission. See, 'A report from Germany – an extract from

    Prospects and Risks of Gene Technology: The Report of the Enquete Commission to the Bundestag of the Federal Republic of Germany', Bioethics vol.2 (1988), pp.256-263.
6   On the matters of disability, health, discrimination and abortion see e.g. the debate, S. Vehmas (1999), 'Discriminative assumptions of utilitarian bioethics regarding individuals with intellectual disabilities', *Disability and Society* vol.14, pp.37-52; R. Rhodes (1999), 'Abortion and assent', *Cambridge Quarterly of Healthcare Ethics* vol.8, pp.416-427; M. Häyry (2001), 'Abortion, disability, assent and consent', *Cambridge Quarterly of Healthcare Ethics* vol.10, pp.79-87.

References

Davis, D.S. (1997), 'Genetic dilemmas and the child's right to an open future', *Hastings Centre Report*, vol.27, pp.7-15.

Feinberg, J. (1992), 'The child's right to an open future', in *Freedom & Fulfilment*, Princeton, Princeton University Press, pp.76-97.

Chapter 5

The Fear of Playing God

Duncan Richter

The previous chapters have been concerned with genetic selection. In this chapter, I turn to the issue of creation. This is possibly even more controversial, especially where the issues of cloning and genetic engineering are concerned. The philosopher Ronald Dworkin has recently argued, in connection to such possibilities, that we should not be afraid to play God.[1] Dworkin argues persuasively that much of the opposition to human cloning arises from such a fear. Less persuasively, he suggests that this fear is misplaced and that in its stead should be a brave rising to the challenge that new scientific techniques pose to mistaken traditional moral thinking. It is mistaken, he says, because it rests on certain factual presuppositions that we can now see to be false. In this chapter I argue that such thinking cannot be a mistake in any straightforward sense and that, even though the research Dworkin supports should go ahead, a certain caution, if not outright fear, is entirely appropriate and potentially beneficial.

If, on religious grounds, a person holds that creating human life is a job for God (and God's gift of sex) only, then this is not a mistake that can be proved false by scientific progress. The question is one of value all the way down, not of fact. The facts about what we cannot change have altered with new technology, but any beliefs about what we ought not to tamper with need not change with them. '[W]e have found', Dworkin says, 'that some of the most basic presuppositions of [our contemporary] values are mistaken'.[2] This may or may not be true. What we *have* found, and presumably, therefore, what Dworkin has in mind, is that we can change some things that we believed previously could not be changed. It seems to me rather hard, though, to be sure just what popular values presuppose, or even what these values are. Indeed, Dworkin himself has worked hard to unearth the real beliefs that lie behind popular statements on the ethics of abortion, euthanasia, and genetic engineering. Certainly, if these values presuppose anything about what science can achieve, such facts might have to do with what is achievable without new technology, rather than what is achievable with any and all future technological developments. Recent advances in biology do not in themselves show traditional morality to be mistaken in any way. The facts, or what we took to be the facts, are no longer true. The same need not be true for our values. Perhaps Dworkin would accept this point and simply modify his choice of words, so I will say no more about it.

More importantly, Dworkin's insightful analysis of the psychology of the fear of playing God points to further dangers that he appears not to see. Dworkin develops the idea that genetic engineering shifts the boundary between chance and choice, between what is simply given and what can be had through human endeavour. This, he rightly observes, is unsettling morally. But, because of all the potential benefits of the new genetics, we should not allow this fear to stop us moving forward.

I agree, but argue that we should do so slowly, for both obvious practical reasons and less obvious philosophical reasons. The most obvious reason for caution is that we do not yet know enough to be able to, say, clone human beings safely, without severe risk of producing deformities, for instance. The less obvious reason for caution is that in unsettling traditional conceptions of what human life is we are, potentially, upsetting the whole applecart of ethics and respect for human life. Roughly speaking, it is up to us how we define human life and human rights. These are not scientific or wholly objective questions. But if we change our definitions too quickly or too often then they are unlikely to be accepted or to become entrenched in our behaviour. In Wittgensteinian terms, if we change the human life form too drastically, we risk undermining our form of life and the whole underpinnings of our ethics. (What would become of humanism, for instance, if our conception of humanity changed radically?) There is a danger of creating a moral vacuum, or at least a moral state worse than the one we have now. In reality this danger is not too great, but this is thanks in large part to a natural conservatism. Drawing on the work of Wittgenstein, Michael Thompson, and certain communitarian theorists (Charles Taylor, Alasdair MacIntyre, and Patrick Devlin), I will argue that the fear of playing God is a useful brake on what might otherwise be a headlong rush into a new age for both ethics and technology.

Some of the objections to human cloning that are most commonly made can quite easily be countered, Dworkin points out. Consider, for instance, objections based on concerns about potential physical dangers, social injustice, and aesthetics. Dworkin does not dismiss these concerns out of hand. There is a real danger of miscarriages and deformity in any experimental method of human reproduction. There is also a real possibility that cloning might be much more readily available to the rich, or even only to the rich, thus increasing the gap between rich and poor. Finally, there is a genuine possibility that if cloning becomes common there could be significantly less diversity in human appearance and indeed a decrease in the number of girls (or boys) that are born, which is not merely an aesthetic concern, of course.

Nevertheless, as valid as such concerns might be, they cannot account for the depth and width of the opposition to human cloning, Dworkin argues. Any new technology or medical technique brings with it dangers, but also new possibilities. As long as we exercise due care, further research into genetic engineering might well produce fewer physical dangers and deformities, not more. Of course we should be careful, but the results could be very beneficial.

As for social justice, the obvious remedy is some sort of redistribution of wealth to tackle the underlying problem of inequality (if this is accepted as a problem), not a crackdown on medical advances whose benefits might be very expensive.

Thirdly, since people have different tastes, even a world filled with clones would still include some diversity, and a measure of aesthetic conformity is valuable. Most of us hope to conform to common standards of beauty, or at least normality, in appearance. The problem of sex selection is more worrying, but selective abortion for sex has been available for some time in the USA, with no uniform result with regard to the numbers of girls and boys being born. Whether parents prefer to have boys or girls, or have no preference, varies from culture to culture. Dworkin possibly dismisses this concern too lightly, since in the cases of India and China sex selection has produced a significant imbalance in favour of males. Still, he is right, I think, that this is not the main reason why people feel uneasy about genetic engineering.

So why is there such revulsion at the thought of genetic engineering, and of human cloning in particular? Dworkin's conclusion is that such feelings arise from an irrational objection to playing God. This objection is irrational since we interfere with nature ('God's plan') all the time, including matters of life and death. This is what technology and medicine are all about, yet they are not generally condemned as unnatural practices. Perhaps this is not what is ordinarily meant when people talk about 'playing God', but what do they mean? It is not entirely clear.

One possible meaning of 'playing God', and a common fear that relates to genetic engineering, is the prospect of artificially created people, or people-like creatures, being used as slaves or organ banks. It seems to me that using human clones as slaves is so clearly wrong that we have no need to fear it happening. Growing mere organs, though, and using them for transplants seems clearly acceptable. What is much less clear is the ethical status of biological products that fall somewhere between complete clones and mere organs. Our common moral intuitions are silent on such things, since traditional values have never had to consider them. Now we do, and this is a problem that brings us back to what it means to be a human being, and what it means to play God.

What this means, in part at least, surely concerns the natural course of events. This, or what is taken to be the natural course of events, is essential to our conception of what a human being is, as Michael Thompson has argued.[3] As a living organism, a human fetus is the kind of thing that naturally develops in a certain way. It belongs to a different logical category than a pile of body parts, say, or other genetic material with the potential to be put together in the form of a human being. To understand what a fetus is, including that it belongs to the human species, we must look to a wider context. A quotation from Thompson will help to clarify the point:

Lab technicians keep lines of human cells of certain types multiplying in vats for ages; suppose then a lake in South America, one maintained by nature in such a character as the lab solution is by art, and shaken perhaps by frequent earthquakes; and now - it does not matter whether it be by a process of evolution from something else, or a quantum-mechanical accident, or an act of God - something as like as you like to a human cell of the appropriate type appears in that sinister fluid. At some point we will have a race of one-celled vegetative creatures, to be given a Latin binomial name and investigated like any other. This kind is evidently not human-kind, and its mode of reproduction is not the human sort. The division that takes place in the lake has a characteristic, *reproduction of the species*, not exhibited in the vat or flask; yet if we ladle up a bit of the lake and take it back to the lab in New York, no test, however subtle, will ever disclose the difference (1995, pp.273-274).

Identifying a fetus or adult human being as human involves relating it to the natural history of the human species. Piles of body parts or miraculous quasi-human cells have no such natural history. And human natural history involves a certain normal development, which is not just the most common development, as Thompson observes.[4] (The normal number of teeth for a human being is not the average number, for instance.) This natural history, which helps define what a human being is, is being altered by new technology.

Dworkin might not share Thompson's view of nature, but he does recognize the ethical significance of the distinction between what we take to be naturally given and what we regard as ours to determine. Indeed, he goes so far as to suggest that 'the overall structure of our moral experience' depends on this distinction.[5] 'This crucial boundary between chance and choice is the spine of our morality, and any serious shift in that boundary is seriously dislocating'.[6] If we change the borderline between what we inescapably are – by chance or the will of God – and what we make ourselves – for good or ill – then we risk dislocating, or perhaps even breaking, this ethical backbone. Dworkin distances himself somewhat from this claim by calling it a hypothesis that he merely invites us to suppose correct, but I think it is correct, and he seems to too.

Dworkin gives several examples of ways in which the boundary between chance and choice plays a key role in our ethics. Ideas about the normal length of human life fundamentally shape the way we think about what it is to have a good life. Traditional ethics have been challenged and stretched by improvements in doctors' ability to keep patients alive and by soldiers' ability to kill large numbers of the enemy. Now the science of genetics confronts us with a new challenge, overturning ancient, entrenched beliefs about 'the brain and body that furnishes for each of us his material substrate' which 'has long been the absolute paradigm of what is both devastatingly important to us and, in its initial condition, beyond our power to alter and therefore beyond the scope of our responsibility...'.[7] It is this issue of responsibility that is of fundamental importance, Dworkin suggests. His hypothesis is not that we *should* significantly change our ideas about who is responsible for what, but that in fact many of us do fear, perhaps not very consciously or articulately, that if we let go of old ideas about responsibility we might fail to grip and hold onto any adequate new one. It is not that morality, right and wrong, will disappear. Dworkin implies that this could not happen ('it would be a serious confusion' to think that morality itself is being challenged, he says).[8] However, he does seem to believe that our *grip* on morality might be lost and that we could find ourselves in 'a kind of moral free-fall'.[9]

Even if this hypothesis is correct (as Dworkin appears to believe, but does not actually claim), this fact does not justify the revulsion felt at the thought of genetic engineering. This is the point Dworkin most wants to make. What we face is a challenge, he says, not a reason to turn back. This challenge must be taken up, not shied away from, 'because the alternative is an irresponsible cowardice in the face of the unknown'.[10]

I think that Dworkin is right to take popular moral intuitions seriously. Whether fully explicable or not, we write off these deep feelings at our peril. As Charles Taylor says, 'My perspective is defined by the moral intuitions I have, by what I am morally moved by. If I abstract from this, I become incapable of understanding any moral argument at all (1989, p.73)'.

Taylor argues that it is pathological to have no sense of what is incomparably important. Without such a sense one simply will be unable to grasp any moral concept. For many people, as Dworkin implies, our physical being is incomparably or 'devastatingly' important. The same could be said of the distinction between what fate hands us and what we create for ourselves. Interference with such fundamentally important matters should not be ruled out *a priori* – the interference might be very useful – but it should not be undertaken lightly. What matters deeply to people is important if for no other reason than precisely that it matters deeply to people, and we should dabble with it carefully, if at all.

This point can be taken too far, though. Patrick Devlin, for example, has argued not only that we need deeply held beliefs but that we need to hold these beliefs in common with others.[11] On these grounds he argues that the law should forbid acts – whatever they might be – that are deeply distasteful to the vast majority of people in a given society. Unfortunately it is unclear just what the moral needs of people are, and Devlin's theory might seem to defend all manner of deep but evil bigotry. Nevertheless, Devlin's view, which is discussed more fully by Matti Häyry in the next chapter, cannot easily be dismissed by anyone who accepts Taylor's belief that nonrational feelings are essential elements in ethical thinking. The natural conclusion to draw seems to be that we should indeed take such feelings seriously – however abhorrent or superstitious they might be – but that this does not justify arch-conservative legislation (of the kind Devlin advocates against gay sex and prostitution, and that might be advocated against research in genetics) absolutely prohibiting behaviour that goes against those feelings. We should not refuse to 'play God', but we should proceed with trepidation. This fear is something to be struggled through, not cast lightly aside.

If our deepest values or beliefs about ethics shift then we run the risk of being unable to make sense of life. Alasdair MacIntyre says that:

> When someone complains – as do some of those who attempt or commit suicide – that his or her life is meaningless, he or she is often and perhaps characteristically complaining that the narrative of their life has become unintelligible to them, that it lacks any point, any movement towards a climax or a *telos* (1984, p.217).

He describes people like this as 'unscripted, anxious stutterers in their actions as in their words (1984, p.216)'.

Serious changes in how human beings are created or develop will change our conception of what it is to be a human being, and perhaps of the degree to which we are creatures (of God) or artifacts. If some of our most fundamental beliefs change too quickly, or have rapidly to be abandoned, then we rightly fear the consequences. As Wittgenstein says in *On Certainty* §616: 'Why, would it be *unthinkable* that I should stay in the saddle however much the facts bucked? (1979)'. It is not unthinkable, and falling out of the ethical saddle is not a fate to be wished. So we should try to ensure that the facts do not buck too much, if at all. Change should be gradual, in other words. Otherwise, in a worst-case scenario, life itself might come to seem meaningless. At the very least, more realistically, ethics might start to seem less meaningful, less important.

Dworkin then is not wrong to focus on the fear of playing God, nor to argue that research should be allowed to go ahead despite this fear. If he believes that such fear is misplaced, though, like an irrational superstition, then he is wrong. For the non-pathological, such fear is entirely natural, if not inevitable, and should serve usefully to slow the rate of change, so that the facts about what we can do evolve or develop, instead of bucking dangerously. It is not only that technology can progress faster than our ability to predict its effects, but also, and perhaps more importantly, that significant moral adjustments will have to be made to our ideas about what it means to be human as science and technology change the physical limits on human beings. Our moral psychology moves quite slowly, or else risks running off the rails. A fear of the changes that technology can bring, then, is both natural and good.[12]

Notes

1   In a paper entitled 'Playing God'. Dworkin's paper exists in multiple forms at the time of writing. It was originally presented at a conference on 'Genetics, Identity and Justice' held by the 21st Century Trust. An edited version was then published in *Prospect* magazine, and it is currently being revised for publication in a forthcoming book of essays on equality (Harvard University Press). My comments will refer to both the *Prospect* version (hereafter referred to as P) and a draft of the latest version, whose pagination is doubtless unique to a copy Professor Dworkin kindly sent to me (hereafter U).

2   Dworkin U, p.36.

3   See Thompson (1995), pp.273-274.

4   Ibid., p.284, '[A]lthough "the mayfly" breeds shortly before dying, *most* mayflies die long before breeding. If the description of the "life-cycle" of the monarch butterfly told us "what mostly happens", then it would soon be unnecessary to visit that strange Mexican valley in order to wade knee-deep among them'.

5   Dworkin P, p.40.

6   Ibid., p.41.

7   Dworkin U, p.34.

8   Ibid., p.36.

9   Ibid.

10 Dworkin P, p.41.

11 See, for instance, Patrick Devlin (1965), *The Enforcement of Morals*, Oxford, Oxford University Press.

12 I am grateful to Stephanie Wilkinson, Brenda Almond and Michael Parker for a number of helpful suggestions made in response to an earlier draft of this paper.

References

McIntyre, A. (1984), *After Virtue*, Notre Dame, Indiana, University of Notre Dame Press.
Taylor, C. (1989), *Sources of the Self*, Cambridge, Massachusetts, Harvard University Press.
Thompson, M. (1995), 'The Representation of Life', in Rosalind Hursthouse, Gavin Lawrence and Warren Quinn (eds), *Virtues and Reasons: Philippa Foot and Moral Theory*, Oxford, Clarendon Press.
Wittgenstein, L. (1979), *On Certainty*, G.E.M. Anscombe and G.H. Von Wright (eds), translated by Denis Paul and G.E.M. Anscombe, Oxford, Basil Blackwell.

Chapter 6

Deeply Felt Disgust – A Devlinian Objection to Cloning Humans

Matti Häyry

The idea of cloning adult human beings often gives rise to objections involving mad dictators producing copies of themselves, or deranged billionaires who want to live forever. But what about situations where we can more readily understand and accept the reasons for creating a clone?

Consider, for instance, the case of parents who have just lost their healthy, newborn child in a freak accident *and* who have recently found out that they cannot have any more children of their own by the more traditional methods of reproduction. They have not stored gametes or frozen embryos, with which they could start a new pregnancy. But they are devastated by the loss of the baby and desperate to have a child whom they could call biologically their own. In these circumstances, would it be wrong of the parents to ask genetic engineers to help them? The experts could seize a somatic cell, still alive for a while, from the infant's body, and make a genetic copy of the lost child. They could clone an embryo which could then be implanted in the mother's uterus or that of a surrogate. Would it be wrong of the parents to want to do this? And would it be wrong of genetic engineers to assist them, assuming that it would be technologically possible?

Arguments against cloning

The most important arguments against cloning human beings who already exist include the following.

First, cloning can be harmful or risky to the clone. This argument is supported by the recent finding that the cells of mammal clones age rapidly. This indicates that there can be a limit to the dividing powers of living cells. But this fact does not necessarily provide us with a reason against cloning newborn infants – their cells are young and can be expected to retain the vitality needed for a 'normal' human development.

Secondly, cloning can be regarded as 'unnatural' or otherwise 'intrinsically immoral'. The best sense I have been able to make of these arguments is within the context of 'personhood'. It can be maintained that individuals produced by cloning would not be *persons* in the full sense of the term because their origin is unnatural. Genetic engineers would, by cloning human beings, play God or otherwise transgress the limits of morality.

I have examined these arguments with Tuija Takala and will not return to them in detail here.[1] Briefly, our findings were the following. It could be wrong to clone adult human beings because the new individuals would, to some extent, be forced to duplicate the lives of their individual parents. But whatever the merits of this view are, it cannot be applied to the case of newborn infants. Their lives have in no sense been pre-lived, and their status as unique and distinct persons remains, therefore, intact.

Thirdly, however, cloning humans can be regarded as offensive to people's feelings and sensitivities. This is the line of argument I will study here in the light of the ideas Lord Patrick Devlin presented in his classic lecture 'The Enforcement of Morals' – which was critically discussed by such eminent philosophers of law as H.L.A. Hart and Ronald Dworkin in the 1960s and 1970s.

The Wolfenden Committee

Let me begin by setting the scene for Devlin's lecture.

In 1954, a Committee was appointed in England to review the laws concerning prostitution and homosexuality (Report of the Committee, 1957). Three years later the Committee, chaired by John Wolfenden, published their report, where they recommended reforms in both areas. The normative starting point for the Committee's work was the distinction made by John Stuart Mill between private and public spheres of morality, or actions which are 'self-regarding' and actions which are 'other-regarding' (Mill, 1859). They reported:

> [The] function of the criminal law [...] is to preserve public order and decency, to protect the citizen from what is offensive or injurious, and to provide sufficient safeguards against exploitation and corruption of others, particularly those who are specially vulnerable because they are young, weak in body or mind, inexperienced, or in a state of special physical, official or economic dependence. (Report of the Committee, 1957, para.13)

For the sake of 'public order and decency', the Committee proposed that prostitution should not be allowed out in the streets – this would be a nuisance to others, to those who are not involved in the business. They also contended that pimping and brothel-keeping should be penalised, because these are potential sources of economic exploitation.

When it comes to homosexual practices and more discreet and direct forms of prostitution, however, the Committee adopted a more lenient view. Since 'private immorality should not be the concern of the criminal law' (Report of the Committee, 1957, para.224), it is not, according to the members of the Committee;

the function of the law to intervene in the private lives of citizens, or to seek to enforce any particular pattern of behaviour, further than is necessary to carry out the purposes we have outlined. (Ibid., para.13)

Drawing on the 'importance which society and the law ought to give to individual freedom of choice and action in matters of private morality', the Committee concluded that laws banning homosexual practices between consenting men should be abolished (lesbianism was not a criminal offence to begin with), and that unobtrusive, nonexploitive forms of prostitution should continue to be untouched by law (Ibid., para.62).

The enforcement of morals

Devlin attacked the Wolfenden Committee report in an honorary lecture on jurisprudence presented to the British Academy in 1959 (Devlin, 1959). Assuming the role of a judge who must pass sentences in a criminal court, he argued that there are acts of 'private immorality' which the law should not view indifferently. The idea of crime, he maintained, should somehow be connected to the idea of sin, or to 'transgression against divine law or the principles of morality' (Ibid., p.3). He wrote:

As a judge who administers the criminal law [...] I should feel handicapped in my task if I thought that I was addressing an audience which had no sense of sin or which thought of crime as something quite different. (Devlin, 1959, p.3)

As examples of cases where the English legal system already recognised the validity of basic moral principles in 'private' matters, he cited the laws forbidding voluntary euthanasia, suicide, attempted suicide, suicide pacts, duelling, abortion, and incest between brother and sister (Ibid., p.4). If the only point of criminal legislation were the protection of individuals, Devlin argued, these laws would not exist. The only way to justify them is by reference to a moral principle.

Despite his appeals to the idea of sin, Devlin did not think that religious arguments could be employed to justify the use of moral principles in criminal legislation. Many Western nations, including England, have ceased to enforce Christian beliefs, showing a lack of appreciation towards the religious basis of their cultures and societies. Devlin believed, accordingly, that, while English law has as its basis the Judaeo-Christian tradition, a more secular justification is needed here, and this he found in the intersection of outraged feelings and the viability of the nation.

Devlin argued that controversial practices can be ethically condemned, and even banned by law, if they provoke certain strong negative feelings in the general public. He did not, however, claim that any immediate reaction by the person in the street would justify legal restrictions. His argument was that feelings can be allowed to guide legislation only if they are experienced (also) by individuals who are calm and appreciate the demands of reason and common sense, and even then only if these feelings reflect the basis of social life in a nation.

There are, of course, other readings of Devlin's work, and I will present some of them further on. But the view I am going to present here is the most favourable interpretation I can think of.

Disgust as a sign

Devlin's analysis can be seen to proceed in three stages. The first of these is formulated in the lecture as follows:

> I do not think one can ignore disgust if it is deeply felt and not manufactured. Its presence is a good indication that the bounds of toleration are being reached. Not everything is to be tolerated. No society can do without intolerance, indignation, and disgust; they are the forces behind the moral law [...]. (Ibid., p.17)

In this widely cited passage Devlin does *not* necessarily say, as many commentators have thought, that if a practice is disgusting to a certain percentage of self-righteous citizens, they should feel free to ban it at will. The message here can be, more moderately, that 'intolerance, indignation, and disgust' can be *signs* of something which should be further investigated by lawyers, ethicists, and philosophers of law. And even this is true only if the feelings in question have not been 'manufactured', presumably by self-serving politicians and the like.

'Disgusting' versus 'vicious'

The second stage of Devlin's argument can be seen to offer a preliminary test for the assessment of actions which give rise to disgust:

> We should ask ourselves in the first instance whether, looking at [the practice in question] calmly and dispassionately, we regard it as a vice so abominable that its mere presence is an offence. If that is the genuine feeling of the society in which we live, I do not see how society can be denied the right to eradicate it. (Ibid., p.17)

Since Devlin used the expression 'the genuine feeling of *the society in which we live*', it is perhaps safe to assume that he did not intend his own emotions to reign universally. In other words, he seemed to recognize the fact that feelings can vary from one location to another, and he thus restricted the power of any given feeling to the community where it is experienced.

Even so, his position is controversial. What if the 'mere presence' of Jewish bankers were 'an offence' to the calm and dispassionate citizens of a particular nation? Would that justify the eradication of Jewish banking activities?

I believe that Devlin could have rejected this implication only by focusing on the concept of 'vice' in the quoted passage. Simple emotions lead to immoral actions. To prevent this, a more profound view of the workings of society is needed. And this can perhaps be developed by making virtues and vices the cornerstones of social life.

Disgust, vice, and social life

Accordingly, Devlin's third step was, or can be read to have been, to explain the moral force of intolerance and disgust by an appeal to social stability. He maintained that these feelings indicate the boundaries of public morality, which we must not overstep if we want to keep our society viable. He supported this idea by explaining what the institution of monogamous marriage meant to his own nation:

> In England we believe in the Christian idea of marriage and therefore adopt monogamy as a moral principle. Consequently the Christian institution of marriage has become the basis of family life and so part of the structure of our society. It is there not because it is Christian. It has got there because it is Christian, but it remains there because it is built into the house in which we live and could not be removed without bringing it down. (Ibid., p.9)

This means, if I have understood correctly what Devlin was saying, that the idea of polygamy was disgusting to the English mind of the late 1950s, because people somehow instinctively knew that its acceptance would have signalled the end of British society as they knew it. And since they had the right to defend their cultural heritage and their traditional way of life, they could not have been 'denied the right to eradicate' the offensive practice.

In a sense which is not entirely trivial, Devlin was probably right. New practices were eventually condoned, and British society is not what it used to be any more. This means that tolerance has brought about (or at least accommodated itself to) changes, as he predicted. What the normative implications of this fact are, is another matter. Many believe that the changes have been for the good. Apparently, Devlin would have thought differently. I will return to the normative significance of social changes shortly.

Anyway, armed with such ideas about the structure of society, Devlin could have argued that Jewish bankers have never been persecuted in Britain, because their activities could never have been offensive to the liberal English mind. If their fate has been grimmer in other countries, this shows, if anything, the moral inferiority of those societies.

The tyranny of the man in the Clapham omnibus?

In order to see the full implications for cloning human beings of the Devlinian view, it is necessary to examine some of the main critiques of his ideas. Ingenious as these critiques are, I believe that they are misleading, although Devlin's choice of words did offer them some justification.

In his account of the role of 'intolerance, indignation, and disgust', Devlin stated that the true lawgiver should be the reasonable (as opposed to the abstractly rational) man, or, in terms used by English jurisprudents of his time, 'the man in the Clapham omnibus' (Ibid., p.15). This expression evoked two reactions, which have remained authoritative in liberal circles. In an early criticism of Devlin, H.L.A. Hart, while commending the democratic appeal of the 'reasonable man' approach, wrote:

> [I]t is fatally easy to confuse the democratic principle that power should be in the hands of the majority with the utterly different claim that the majority with power in their hands need respect no limits. Certainly there is a special risk in a democracy that the majority may dictate how all should live. [...] But loyalty to democratic principles does not require us to maximize this risk: yet this is what we shall do if we mount the man in the street on the top of the Clapham omnibus and tell him that if only he feels sick enough about what other people do in private to demand its suppression by law no theoretical criticism can be made of his demand. (Hart, 1959, pp.87-88)

And Ronald Dworkin later joined Hart in complaining that Devlin;

> without offering evidence that homosexuality presents any danger at all to society's existence, [...] concludes that if our society hates homosexuality enough it is justified in outlawing it, [...] because of the danger the practice presents to society's existence. (Dworkin, 1977, p.246)

These contributions carved in stone the 'liberal' reading that, defying both logic and rational ethics, Devlin wanted to ban all practices which can be seen as disgusting by the 'moral majority'.

Had this been the message Devlin tried to convey, his contribution to the cloning debate would be simple and short-lived. Some people could, by an appeal to his views, claim that cloning should be prohibited as an offence to their sensibilities, and, consequently, to the sensibilities of 'reasonable men'. And others could counter this claim by arguing that feelings do not or cannot justify the proposed legal restrictions.

If, however, Devlin's view contains the three layers I have described, it is misguided to accuse him, as Hart and Dworkin did, of relying on people's immediate reactions. The intertwined facts that 'our society hates homosexuality', and that the 'reasonable man' confirms this emotional judgement only suggest that our society *can* be threatened by the practice and that the matter should be looked into more closely.

A corollary of this view is that disgust, however deeply felt, does not really do any decisive normative work in Devlin's model. It is only a sign, and must be regarded as such. The true justification for banning distasteful activities is that they somehow damage the structure of society.

What kind of injury?

In a later, more balanced, discussion of Devlin's principles, Hart distinguished between two separate theses concerning immorality and the law (Hart, 1963). According to the extreme thesis, 'morality as such' must be protected by law whenever righteous citizens feel that it is threatened by a practice which is disgusting. This is the 'Clapham omnibus' approach, with its obvious flaws. But a more moderate reading of Devlin's views also offered itself to Hart. Shortly after the passage stating that 'intolerance, indignation and disgust are the forces behind the moral law', Devlin wrote:

> It is the power of common sense and not the power of reason that is behind the judgements of society. But before a society can put a practice beyond the limits of tolerance there must be a deliberate judgement that the practice is injurious to society. (1965, op. cit. p.120)

Passages like this presumably made Hart see that the basis for Devlin's model can, in theory, also be found in the harm or injury which can befall society if its laws are recklessly altered. According to the moderate thesis, morality can be legitimately protected if its collapse would be injurious or harmful.

Hart argued that the distinction between the two theses reveals the dilemma facing Devlin's doctrine. If morality is to be safeguarded 'as such', mob rule will follow, and this is not good. But if, on the other hand, morality can be rightfully protected only if failing to do so would be harmful, then Devlin's views cannot be distinguished from Mill's liberalism which he had set out to refute.

Hart's critique, then, is that Devlin's model is either against Mill or acceptable, but not both. It is acceptable if deeply felt disgust is seen as a sign of such immorality that its approval would harm innocent people. But since the ultimate criterion here is harmfulness, Hart concluded, the model is utilitarian and inseparable from Mill's system.

Liberty or morality?

While Hart may have been mostly right in what he was arguing, Devlin's views can, nevertheless, be distinguished from the utilitarian ideals advocated by Mill – and, perhaps, by the Wolfenden Committee. It is one thing to say that practices are directly harmful to identifiable individuals and groups, such as prostitutes, young and impressionable boys, or individuals who have been produced by cloning. Yet it is another thing to draw attention to the indirect harm inflicted on members of existing communities by radical changes in legislation and social life.

The important question is, are societies allowed to change at all in Devlin's model? If the answer is no, then his doctrine can be accused of being unrealistic. Societies have not always remained the same, and arguably some past developments have made people's lives better, not worse. Devlin's views on this point are not entirely clear. But in an essay titled 'Mill on Liberty in Morals' he outlined the history of legislative morality in an illuminating way.

In *On Liberty*, Mill maintained that the fallibility of rulers provides a sufficient reason for allowing changes in law and morality. His example was Marcus Aurelius, who could see Christianity only as a force which would destroy the morality he was brought up to respect (Mill, 1996, pp.28-29). But since history shows, according to Mill, that the morality generated by Christianity was superior to the Roman ethos, lawgivers should think twice before they try to supress new ways of thinking. More particularly, Mill thought that his ideal of liberty should be assumed by the enlightened legislators of his own time.

Devlin agreed that Christian morality was in its time superior to the Roman law, and he went on to sketch the changes which have, or could have, ensued. He wrote:

> In our societies we believe in the advance of man towards a goal and this belief is the mainspring of our morals. We believe that at some time in the history of mankind, whether on a sudden by a divine stroke or imperceptibly in evolution over millennia, there were extracted from the chaos of the primeval mind concepts of justice, benevolence, mercy, continence, and others of that ilk which we call virtues. The distinction between virtue and vice, between good and evil so far as it affects our actions is what morals are about. (Devlin, 1964, p.120)

In the Middle Ages, when religion was strong in the minds of people, there was a 'common agreement about the end of man' (Devlin, 1965, op. cit. p.120). This, according to Devlin, is what a 'common religious faith' means (Ibid.). In modern times, this has been replaced by a 'common agreement about the way he [man] should go', which is the mark of a 'common moral faith' (Ibid.). Although we have given up the belief in one unified religion, we are still left with the faith in morals, that is, in the distinction between virtue and vice, or 'in the *direction* we are all travelling to'.[2] And this is what Millian liberals are denying, or trying to deprive us of, by insisting that morals must not be enforced by law.

Reform or stability?

The obvious Millian reply is that the 'direction we are all travelling to' is the direction of liberty. We can define as virtuous those actions which are not injurious to others, and as vicious those actions which are. Vice can be censured, as our moral faith demands, while we can insist on banning only activities which are harmful. Devlin himself wrote in *The Enforcement of Morals* that the 'limits of tolerance shift', and that it 'may be that over-all tolerance is increasing', as the 'pressure of human mind, always seeking greater freedom of thought, is outwards against the bonds of society forcing their gradual relaxation' (Devlin, 1965, p.18). So why not see the Millian society as the next logical step?

Devlin's answer seems to be that extreme liberalism could indeed be the next step, but that legislators cannot be the ones to bring about the change. The reason for this is that today's legislators can hardly hope to be wiser than Marcus Aurelius was. They do not know what lies in the future, and they must therefore do what *they* think is *right*. He wrote:

> To admit that we are not infallible is not to admit that we are always wrong. What we believe to be evil may indeed be evil and we cannot for ever condemn ourselves to inactivity against evil because of the chance that we may by mistake destroy good. For better or worse the law-maker must act according to his lights and he cannot therefore accept Mill's doctrine as practicable even if as an ideal he thought it to be desirable. (Devlin, 1965, p.123)

The best sense I can make of this is that legislators must enforce the morality they see as beneficial to society, provided that the immediate reactions of the community are on their side. These reactions – intolerance, indignation and disgust – do not in the final analysis *prove* that a practice is immoral, but they show where the bounds of tolerance presently lie.

This means that, in Devlin's model, lawmakers should not be ahead of their time and perhaps that they should not fall too far behind either. In retrospect, for instance, the British society of the 1950s could not tolerate homosexual practices between consenting men, but the situation has now changed. This is why the laws were amended. But if Devlin was right, it would have been wrong of the legislators to interfere with the process, because it is safer that the law is slow to change.

As far as I can see, the rational debate between Devlin and his opponents comes to an end here. Millian reformists want the laws to change society, Devlinian conservatives want them to change only with society. Proponents of Mill see freedom as the absence of restrictions and allow constraints only if our actions harm others. Devlin defined a free society differently, and contended that excessive liberty would make 'society intolerable for most of us' (Ibid.). In what follows I will adopt, for argument's sake, the Devlinian view, to see what its implications for cloning would be. (The Millian view would probably favor liberty in the case of the newborn, but that is an issue which must be examined separately.)

Devlin's argument in a nutshell

To summarise, Devlin's three steps for banning offensive practices are, according to my interpretation, the following:

1   Spontaneous and widely shared feelings of disgust indicate something that should be looked into by law-makers.
2   If these feelings persist under a cool and impassionate analysis, and certain practices are deemed to be truly vicious, the claim that these feelings reflect society's moral fibre is strong and worthy of careful examination.
3   If these feelings can be shown to correspond with the core of the society's way of life and with its most basic beliefs, the practices they censure can be justifiably banned by the laws of that society, because they would harm the society as a moral entity.

My question is, do these points justify a legal ban on cloning in all circumstances? My answer is that I doubt it. But let me proceed one step at a time.

Cloning and slow legal change?

The Devlinian approach is still open to one objection which must be addressed to clarify the picture. It is that laws on cloning did not exist in most countries before the birth of Dolly. If legislators are not allowed to bring about changes, what could justify their interference in this new area?

The answer to this question, if anyone would care to pose it, probably is that the moral principles which prohibit abortion, euthanasia and duelling, and which have already been recognized in Western legal systems, also support the ban on cloning human beings. New technologies cannot have legal immunity just because they have emerged after the legislation concerning similar activities has been passed. The slowness of legal change is supposed to put brakes on the expansion of tolerance, not to license potentially intolerable practices which have only recently been invented.

This would presumably also be the Devlinian line of argument concerning abortion, euthanasia and duelling, which have only been legally banned since the nineteenth century. These prohibitions were based on the principle of the sanctity of life, which is a part of the Western cultural heritage and which has needed the support of the law in recent times due to developments in medicine, etiquette and weapons technology.

Cloning and immediate disgust

How, then, should Devlin's three points be applied to the case of cloning? First, is cloning human beings a practice which evokes, spontaneously, feelings of 'intolerance, indignation, and disgust' in our contemporary societies? The answer is not as straightforward as the opponents of cloning would like to think.

True, the idea of cloning humans *in general* may seem disgusting, as evidenced by the reactions to the news regarding Dolly the sheep (National Bioethics

Advisory Commission, 1997). But what about the case where genetic engineering would be the only way to 'save' the lost baby of the unfortunate parents in my example? I suspect that many people would say that this is different – the agony of the parents is real and concrete, and if it can be alleviated by using new technologies, this should be done.

The situation is, by the way, similar in Devlin's original context, in the context of banning homosexuality. Even people who think that homosexual practices are disgusting *in general* may have different views of particular cases. The imprisonment of Oscar Wilde for his 'offences' does not always seem right even to persons who are happy to condemn his sexual orientation on a more general level. And parents who advocate the imprisonment of 'sodomites' may change their minds if their own son turns out to be one of the offenders.

Cloning considered 'calmly and dispassionately'

Paradoxically, the second step in Devlin's argument, the requirement of calm and dispassionate examination, yields more restrictive results. At least some scientists, philosophers and theologians who have considered things carefully in the light of biology, ethics and religion have concluded that the prohibition of cloning humans ought to be absolute.[3] How can this be explained, and what does it mean in the Devlinian framework?

The answer takes us back to Devlin's first point and to the possibility of 'manufacturing' disgust. How spontaneous should the negative feelings be? Would Devlin have ruled out outrage if it had been the result of scientific, philosophical or theological indoctrination? I believe that the answer must be 'yes', since his own primary aim was to reject the Millian philosophical model where only 'harmful' actions can be legally banned. Furthermore, normative doctrines cannot be divided into those that are acceptable and those that are not, as Devlin's argument centres on concrete emotions, as opposed to any abstract theories.

The views of scientists, philosophers and theologians cannot, therefore, override the immediate reactions of the general public. Disgust which is felt only within a particular world view or moral doctrine is, in Devlin's sense, manufactured and, for his purposes, tainted. This means that the possible indignation of ethicists who would like to ban the cloning of babies is as irrelevant as the feelings of Mill's followers who would be disgusted by the prohibition.

Cloning and society

The third and final question is, are our societies seriously threatened by the possibility of cloning? Would the practice of making genetic copies of living human beings alter our ways of life so radically that our governments have the right to prohibit it in the name of social and cultural self-preservation?

Tentatively and cautiously, in the case of cloning adults, maybe yes. We are rather accustomed to the idea that we are all genetically different, with the exception of identical twins. Perhaps dozens of genetically identical individuals would change our societies radically. Family trees would be distorted. Laws concerning inheritance would have to be altered. Criminal investigation would in some cases be more difficult. Genetic discrimination might occur. I am not certain that these would present insurmountable problems, but at least a case against cloning adults can be based on these observations.

It is not, however, clear to me how helping the parents of my example to reproduce their lost infant would pose a threat to social life as we know it. It could, of course, be the thin end of the wedge, or the camel's nose – the legal acceptance of cloning in some situations could lead to its acceptance in others as well. But this is not a serious consideration in Devlin's model. He did, after all, admit that times can change, albeit slowly, and laws with them. The clear implication is that arguments founded on disgust have to be looked at in their historical context. This means that if, in the future, the cloning of even adult human beings is not viewed with indignation any more, then the restrictions can, arguably, be lifted.

Conclusions

I conclude that Devlin's argument cannot be employed to prohibit the cloning of newly born infants if this is the only method by which the parents of a dead baby can have children who carry their own genes. People's spontaneous feelings of disgust are not strong enough to support the ban, and emotions manufactured by ethical theories are inadmissible as evidence. What is more, life in our societies would not be seriously threatened by this exception.

The corollary of this conclusion is that cloning as such is not always wrong, unless other arguments can be found against it. The search for these arguments was not the aim of this paper.

On a more personal note, can I add that I see little point in cloning babies in the first place. The alleviation of agony in my example is marginal, and I think that the money should be allocated to more sensible purposes. But here I have proceeded from what I believe are more widely shared feelings in our contemporary affluent societies than mine are.

Notes

1   M. Häyry and T. Takala 'Cloning, naturalness and personhood', in D.C. Thomasma, D.N. Weisstub, C. Hervé, (eds) *Personhood and Health Care*, Dordrecht, Kluwer Academic Publishers, in print.
2   Devlin (1965). Not a direct quote.
3   See, for example, R. Williamson (1999), 'Human reproductive cloning is unethical because it undermines autonomy, 'Commentary on Savulescu', *Journal of Medical*

Ethics, vol.25, pp.96-97, D. Callahan (1997), 'Cloning: The work not done', *Hastings Center Report,* vol.27(5), pp.18-20, and Pontificia Academia Pro Vita (1997), *Reflexions on Cloning,* Vatican City: Libreria Editrice Vaticana.

References

Devlin, P. (1959), 'The Enforcement of Morals'. Reprinted (as 'Morals and the Criminal Law') in *The Enforcement of Morals* (1965), Oxford, Oxford University Press.

Devlin, P., (1964) 'Mill on Liberty in Morals'. Reprinted in *The Enforcement of Morals,* Oxford, Oxford University Press, 1965.

Dworkin, R. (1977), *Taking Rights Seriously,* Oxford, Oxford University Press.

Hart, H.L.A. (1959), 'Immorality and treason'. Reprinted in R.M. Dworkin (ed.) (1977), *The Philosophy of Law,* Oxford, Oxford University Press.

Hart, H. L. A. (1963), *Law, Liberty and Morality,* Oxford, Oxford University Press.

Mill. J.S., *On Liberty* (1859). Reprinted in *On Liberty and The Subjection of Women,* Ware, Hertfordshire, Wordsworth Classics of World Literature, 1996.

National Bioethics Advisory Commission (1997), *Executive Summary. Cloning Human Beings: The Report and Recommendations of the National Bioethics Advisory Commission,* Rockland, Maryland.

Report of the Committee on Homosexual Offences and Prostitution, Cmd. 247, 1957.

Chapter 7

Genetic Intervention and Personal Identity

Walter Glannon

Introduction

Previous chapters have considered some of the more controversial possibilities offered by the new genetic technologies – selecting embryos for preferred characteristics, genetic engineering for general enhancement reasons, and the cloning of human beings. In this chapter, I start from consideration of what is probably the least controversial use that can be made of these technologies: genetic modification of embryos for *bona fide* medical reasons, and I ask: How does such intervention affect our notion of personal identity? Should we regard it as a matter of helping a continuing person, or does it in fact amount to substituting for one person or possible person another quite different one?

Genetic technology has given us the ability to intervene in the functions of somatic and germ cells to treat, prevent, or even cure genetically caused diseases. Presently, we can add normal copies of genes to cells with defective genes so that the proteins the genes encode will maintain proper cell functioning. It also may become possible to replace malfunctioning genes with normal ones. Both somatic- and germ-cell manipulation have significant metaphysical and moral implications. They can affect the identities of the individuals whose genes are manipulated and can determine who is benefited or harmed by intervening to treat physical and mental disorders with a genetic cause.

I will explore the extent to which genes affect personhood and personal identity, showing that genes as such influence but do not determine who we are and how we persist as the same individuals through time. Then I will argue that the earlier genetic intervention takes place in the development of a human organism, the more likely it will determine that the person who comes into existence from that organism will be distinct from the person who would have existed had the intervention not taken place. In contrast, the later intervention occurs in the life of a person, the more likely it is to preserve the identity of one and the same person. Generally, the former will involve germ-cell intervention, while the later will involve somatic-cell intervention. However, I will present examples to illustrate that in some, particularly mental, genetic disorders, intervention into somatic cells can alter personal identity. This suggests that, in order to be therapeutic and thus benefit persons, genetic intervention must preserve the identity of the individuals who are treated. A further implication of this point is that germ-line intervention cannot appropriately be characterized as therapeutic since, when it occurs at the embryonic stage, no individual exists who could benefit or be harmed by it. I will confine the discussion to genetic prevention and treatment, leaving aside genetic enhancements. The general upshot will be that in all forms of genetic intervention metaphysical and moral issues are inextricably intertwined.

How genes influence biological and personal identity

The particular phenotypic traits caused by the genetic polymorphisms that physically distinguish each of us from other human organisms constitute our biological identity. But the biological identity of a human organism is not equivalent to the psychological identity of a person. The capacity for consciousness and the mental states which makes us persons is generated and sustained by a normally functioning brain. These states also causally depend on the body, which serves as a ground reference for our mental representations of what we perceive in the external world.[1] Still, mental states are not reducible to, in the sense of being completely explained by, the brain and body. The qualitative character of consciousness—*what it is like* to perceive colours or remember an experienced event—cannot be explained in biological terms alone. Moreover, the contents of our mental representations are at least partly determined by features of the social and physical environment in which we exist.

To be a person, one must have the capacity for conscious awareness of one's continued existence over time (Parfit, 1984, p.202). Following the standard psychological continuity account defended by Parfit and others, personal identity consists in the holding of certain relations of psychological connectedness and continuity between and among mental states over periods of time.[2] According to Parfit, connectedness consists in the holding of particular direct links between mental events and states, such as the persistence of beliefs and desires, the connection between an intention and the later act in which it is realized, and the connection between an experience and one's memory of it. These connections can be stronger, holding over shorter periods of time, or weaker, holding over longer periods. Psychological continuity is the ancestral relation of psychological connectedness, consisting in overlapping chains of strong connectedness and extending over longer periods of time than what is involved in particular links between mental states (Ibid., pp.213-4). Unlike connectedness, continuity does not admit of degrees and is a transitive relation. That is, it embodies the truth of the syllogism: If A at time 1 is identical to B at time 2, and if B at time 2 is identical to C at time 3, then A at time 1 is identical to C at time 3.

Because the capacity for mental life and the relations holding between mental states which define personhood and personal identity through time are causally dependent on biological features of human organisms at embryonic and earlier stages, persons are related to their organisms. But persons are metaphysically distinct from their organisms because the capacity for mental life is not an essential property of organisms. Put another way, a person is constituted by a human organism but is not identical to that organism. An entity with a functioning body and brain stem but lacking a functioning cerebral cortex necessary to generate and sustain mentality would be a human organism, but not a person, as in the case of anencephalic infants. Similarly, an individual in a persistent vegetative state with irreversible loss of the capacity for mentality would be a human organism (or human being) but not a person. If we take ourselves to be essentially entities with the capacity for consciousness and other forms of mentality, if these properties are definitive of personhood, and if being a human organism does not entail having this capacity or these properties, then it follows that we are essentially persons rather than human organisms or human beings. Although persons cannot plausibly be separated from their organisms because their defining psychological properties causally depend on biological properties of the body and brain, they are not reducible or identical to their organisms.[3] I will support this claim by considering the role of genes in cell differentiation.

While an increasing number of cells follow a continuous line of development in human organisms from the embryonic stage to further stages, this does not mean that a single individual persists through the entire process. For during this period of development, embryonic cells undergo a continuous process of differentiation into distinct cell, tissue, and organ types. Differentiation implies that the biological features of the organism undergo significant qualitative changes from zygotic and embryonic to later fetal stages. As embryologist C. R. Austin notes, 'the whole embryo *does not* become the fetus—only a small fraction of the embryo is thus involved, the rest of it continuing as the placenta and other auxiliary structures' (Austin, 1989, p.17). Moreover, even if the cerebral cortex is present in rudimentary form in fetuses and has the potential to generate mentality, this does not mean that fetuses become (in the identity-preserving sense of 'become') persons. For, as molecular biologist Lee Silver points out, 'although the cerebral cortex—the eventual seat of human awareness and emotions—has begun to grow, the cells within it are not capable of functioning as nerve cells. They are simply precursors to nerve cells without the ability to send or receive any neurological signals. Further steps of differentiation must occur' (Silver, 1997, p.64).

Cell differentiation is a form of epigenesis. While in strict molecular terms epigenesis is the study of heritable changes in gene expression that occur without a change in DNA sequence, it literally means 'after' or 'over' genes (Wolfe and Matzke, 1999). Successive stages of cell differentiation in the course of an organism's development give rise to new structures with new properties. The genetic code in the zygote or preimplantation embryo only specifies the *general* range of possible phenotypic outcomes in a human organism. It does not determine which *particular* traits will manifest themselves at the end of the process. This is because the genetic code itself cannot account for the interactions between the products of successive stages of development, and because the translation of genetic material into a particular phenotype depends on the particular environment in which development takes place. In considering the process of development from zygote to embryo to full-fledged human organism, the uterine environment is especially pertinent. In the brain, for example, certain genes code for a range of synapses and neurotransmitter levels. But the particular synapses that form and the levels of neurotransmitters mediating between these synapses result from the interaction between genes and the uterine environment during fetal development. All of this suggests that one's genotype (a person's or an organism's genetic make-up) is not identical to one's phenotype (a person's or an organism's observable traits), and that the mentality that makes us persons is determined by neither of these biological types. If genes by themselves do not determine the particular structures and functions of our brains and bodies, and if our brains and bodies do not by themselves determine the content and qualitative character of the mental states that make us persons, then personhood and personal identity are influenced but not determined by genotype and phenotype.

This account of cell differentiation indicates that the mere potential of a zygote or embryo to develop into a person is not enough to establish a relation of identity between these distinct stages of human development. This is precisely because the properties of each successive stage are so different from those of preceding stages. Thus a person never was a zygote or embryo, and these entities do not become persons. A zygote or embryo is a potential person, not in the sense that it becomes a person, but only in the sense that it has the potential to develop the biological structures and functions necessary to generate and sustain the capacity for consciousness and other forms of mentality that essentially define persons.[4] Genetic identity is not personal identity. But manipulation of genes at different stages in the development of a human organism, or in the psychological life of a person, can affect the nature of and the connections between mental states. It can determine whether a set of mental states which persists through time belongs to one person or distinct persons. Let us now examine how different forms of genetic intervention can affect personal identity, as well as how this metaphysical question bears on the moral question of who benefits from such intervention.

Genetic interventions

Once the relations between mental states are formed and become richer over time as one lives longer, significant disruption in the connectedness and continuity of these states is required for personal identity to be altered. Intuitively, in a physical genetic disorder like cystic fibrosis (CF), even if somatic-cell gene therapy at some point in the individual's late childhood or early adolescence restored normal lung and pancreatic function, it is doubtful that this cure would effect a change in the identity of the person. To be sure, these individuals would be different before and after the therapy in the sense that the contents of and the connections between their desires and intentions would change somewhat given the knowledge that they would live longer and would not be physically restricted by the disease. Yet they would not literally become different persons, because their memories of their past experience with the disease would not be lost but would remain with them. The connections between one's experiences and one's memory of them are an essential component of personal identity. Indeed, the backward-looking memories of pain and suffering with the disease might even shape the forward-looking desires and intentions without the disease if, for example, one devoted the rest of one's life to helping others with CF.

In the case of an older child or adolescent receiving somatic-cell gene therapy for CF or some other genetically caused physical disorder, the individual's biological life after the procedure would in important respects be different from their biological life before the procedure. But insofar as only some of the connections between the individual's mental states were thereby affected, there would be one person with one continuous psychological life before and after the therapy. In Parfit's words, 'to say that literally a different person appeared would require a break in the deeper relation of continuity, not just connectedness' (Parfit, 1976, p.103). Recall that continuity involves overlapping chains of strong connectedness. The more robust and unified a set of mental states becomes over time, the more overlapping chains there are of these states. Accordingly, the more radical the changes to these states must be to disrupt psychological continuity and hence personal identity

When a genetic intervention occurs is crucial to the question of whether it will be identity-determining or identity-preserving. The earlier the intervention occurs, the more likely it will determine that the identity of the person who comes into existence as a result of it will be different from the one who would have existed without the intervention. The later it occurs, the more likely it is to preserve the identity of one and the same person. Somatic-cell gene intervention for most physical disorders would preserve identity largely because it would occur after all the body's cells have differentiated, while germ-line genetic intervention for any physical or mental disorder would be identity-determining because it would occur before cell differentiation and thus would affect all the cells in the embryo that would develop into a person. In the first case, there would be a distinct biological life from the time of the genetic intervention; but there would be one continuous psychological life of one person. In the second case, there would be two distinct biological and psychological lives of two distinct human organisms and two distinct people. Yet there are some cases of early somatic-cell intervention which would be identity-determining.

Consider the recently reported successful treatment of two babies, aged 11 and 8 months, for a form of severe combined immune deficiency (SCID) (Cavazzano-Calvo, et al., 2000). Because the biological consequences of the intervention are so significant, and because neither baby had yet to develop an integrated set of psychological properties, the biological properties resulting from the treatment will entail a different set of psychological properties and thus different persons from those that would have existed without the treatment. In contrast, if somatic-cell gene therapy could cure an individual of CF in late childhood or adolescence, then from the time of the therapy we would be considering a distinct biological life but the same psychological life of the same person who existed before the therapy. For he already would have developed an integrated set of psychological properties, and the changes to these properties which the intervention effected would not be so radical as to disrupt psychological continuity. But germ-line intervention at the zygotic or embryonic stage of development would determine distinct biological and psychological lives from the lives that would have existed without the intervention. For at that point no psychological connections could have formed and therefore no person could yet exist.

Similar reasoning applies to the case of a boy with Duchenne muscular dystrophy (DMD). This is a recessive genetic disorder traceable to a mutation on the X chromosome which is transmitted to 50% of males whose mothers carry the mutation. The mutation causes dysfunction of the dystrophin protein, resulting in the gradual weakening of muscles and subsequent respiratory failure and death by around age 20. Presumably, the boy could file a tort of wrongful life against his obstetrician or biological parents, claiming that his life was not worth living and that accordingly they should not have brought him into existence.[5] But he could not hold them responsible or liable for failing to avail themselves of genetic technology that could have replaced the abnormal gene coding for the dysfunctional dystrophin gene with a normal gene in the cells of the embryo from which he developed. For in that case *he* would not have existed. The replacement of the abnormal gene with a normal gene at the germ line before cell differentiation was underway would have meant a completely different set of subsequent biological and psychological properties belonging to a completely different individual. So the child could claim only that the wrong of wrongful life was committed by not terminating the further development of the embryo from which he developed. He could not also claim that he was harmed by his parents' failure to add a normal copy of the crucial gene to prevent him from having the disease. Adding the normal gene would have meant than he would not have existed, and therefore no one would have been harmed.

Significantly, germ-line genetic intervention cannot appropriately be characterized as gene therapy, but rather as prevention of a genetically caused disease. Therapy implies treatment that benefits one by making one better off than one was before the treatment, which requires a comparison between two states of affairs in which the same individual exists.[6] But since at the zygotic and embryonic stages there is no individual who exists with a disease, at that stage of development there is no one who could benefit from the intervention. So it cannot be therapeutic in any plausible sense of the term. Because germ-line intervention is fundamentally a preventive intervention occurring before cell differentiation and therefore before any genetic damage has occurred in cells, only somatic-cell intervention can properly be characterized as 'gene therapy'.[7]

It is important to spell out the moral implications of somatic-cell and germ-line genetic intervention, specifically in terms of how these interventions can benefit or harm (in the case of gene therapy gone awry) persons. Only persons can have interests, since only persons have the mental capacity for desires, beliefs, and intentions necessary for interests. Insofar as benefit and harm result from the satisfaction or defeat of interests, only persons can be benefited or harmed.[8] An individual is benefited when she is made better off than she was or would have been, and is harmed when she is made worse off than she was or would have been. This is not the case for germ-line intervention at earlier stages of human development, however. Since zygotes and embryos do not have any capacity for mentality, they are not identical to persons. And because they lack this capacity that is necessary for interests, zygotes and embryos cannot be benefited or harmed. It follows, then, that no entity at any stage of a developing human organism prior to the emergence of personhood can benefit from or be harmed by the addition, replacement, or deletion of a gene or genes at the germ line.

Nevertheless, because genetic manipulation at these early stages of development can result in effects on the bodies and minds of the people who develop from them, persons can benefit from or be harmed by such manipulation.

These persons would not have interests at the time the manipulation took place, since they would not yet exist. But because the manipulation of a gene, together with its interactions with other genes and environmental factors, can affect the ways in which the genotype translates into the phenotype and results in varying states of mental and physical health or disease, people subsequently can be affected by it. The benefits or harms occur not because, before they existed, the people in question had an interest in not being diseased. Rather, once they exist, they have an interest in not experiencing the pain, suffering, and restricted opportunities entailed by genetically caused diseases.

It seems that what matters here is not so much *who* will or would have to experience the symptoms of genetically caused diseases, but rather *that* someone will or would have to experience them. Put another way, if we were to intervene at some point in the life of a human organism or person to correct a genetic mutation and thereby prevent, cure, or alleviate the symptoms of a disease caused by that mutation, whom it will affect is not as significant as that we intervene in such a way as to prevent or eliminate the disease so that no one would have to experience its harmful effects. The experience of disease can affect the content and phenomenological character of one's mental states and thus affect personal identity. But to the extent that persons are interested in not having mental states of this type, the moral question of benefit, or harm, appears to be at least as important as the metaphysical question of identity. The two questions cannot be separated. Yet cases of genetic intervention to treat cognitive disorders suggest that the metaphysical question is more fundamental than the moral one, and indeed that the very idea of benefit depends on the idea of identity.

Cognitive gene 'therapy' and a paradox about equality

All of the cases that I have discussed thus far involve physical genetic diseases. More difficult to assess is genetic intervention to correct or treat a genetically caused mental disorder at any stage of a person's life. Recently, scientists reported that they were able to manipulate a gene in the brains of mice and thereby enhance their memory, suggesting the possibility of restoring or even improving cognitive capacity through manipulation of the analogous gene or genes in humans (Ya-Ping Tang et al., 1999). Quite apart from the obvious differences between mice and humans, it is simplistic to think that a single gene or gene product could control intelligence, which is a function of complex interactions among different genes, whose functions in turn are affected by the interactions between a human organism and its social and physical environment. Still, subtle alterations in brain biochemistry can affect the nature and content of mental states such as desires, beliefs, intentions, and emotions, which are constituents of personal identity through time. And manipulating one gene that plays a crucial role in cognitive or emotional mental function could affect these states and thus identity. While genetic intervention to treat mental impairment is not likely in the foreseeable future, it is instructive to test our intuitions by considering the respects in which genetic intervention to improve one's cognitive or emotional capacity could affect personal identity.

Whether these sorts of intervention would be identity-preserving or identity-determining would depend on the purpose of the intervention as well as the nature of the disorder in question. If a person were to lose previously normal mental functioning as a result of a stroke, then the purpose of any genetic treatment (involving, say, angiogenesis to restore blood flow and neuronal connections) on the relevant parts of his brain would be to restore him to the level of mental functioning he had before the stroke. While there would be a gap in psychological connectedness and continuity during the period when he was experiencing the effects of the stroke, the intervention ideally would restore connectedness and continuity and hence his identity. On the other hand, if cognitive or affective treatment were performed on someone with moderately severe to severe mental impairment from birth due to a genetic or chromosomal anomaly, such as Fragile X or Down syndrome, then the aim of the treatment would be to raise their level of mental functioning to the level that is normal for persons generally.

In each case, the genetic intervention would have a therapeutic rationale. But it would have a different impact on personal identity. In the first case, the restorative effect of the intervention would re-establish the connections between the normal mental states the person had prior to the stroke with the normal states he would have following the treatment. There would indeed be some disconnectedness and discontinuity between the time of the stroke and the time the treatment restored his normal mental functioning, though, crucially, these would be temporary rather than permanent. Provided that the temporal gap was not too long, the intervention would restore his mental functioning and identity and therefore would appropriately be called 'therapy'. In the second case, the nature and contents of the individual's mental states would be radically different before and after the genetic intervention and therefore the genetic intervention would mean that the original individual with the mental disorder became a distinct person. But if this were the case, then the intervention could not be therapeutic. For the person who presumably benefited from it would no longer exist. The treatment for the mental disorder would radically alter the mental states and thus the identity of the person who had the disorder. Notably, this problem would not arise in the case of the treatment of the SCID babies mentioned earlier. At the time of the intervention, they would lack a sufficiently integrated set of psychological properties to be considered full-fledged persons.

The intervention in the stroke case could be defended on grounds of beneficence and justice. By restoring the person to the level of mental and physical functioning he had before the stroke, we would be benefiting him by making him better off than he otherwise would have been by having to live with the adverse effects of the stroke on his physical and cognitive functioning. Moreover, correcting the dysfunction would restore him to the level where he had the same opportunities as other people to undertake and complete projects within a life plan of his own making.[9]

On the other hand, if we could deliver a gene or genes into the brain of a severely cognitively or affectively disabled individual and dramatically raise their mental functioning to a normal level, then we would not benefit *this* person. They could not be made better off because the change in their mental states would alter their identity. Again, the intervention would not be therapeutic. Presumably, the justice requirement would offer stronger reasons for improving the mentally disabled individual's cognitive and affective capacities through genetic means. An individual should have opportunities for projects and achievements of which he is deprived owing to his mental disability, opportunities equal to those possessed by people with normal mental functioning. Even here, though, the difference in identity before and after the intervention suggests that the justice requirement would pertain more to the level of cognitive and affective capacity than to the particular persons who have or lack these capacitie. It would not matter morally, one might argue, that a particular cognitively or affectively disabled person became a different person following genetic intervention, only that some persons had the same level of mental functioning and the same opportunities for achievement as other persons.

This suggests a utilitarian argument for justice. That is, raising the aggregate level of mental functioning across all people matters morally more than the level of mental functioning of particular people. Yet, when we specify the justice requirement, we ordinarily assume that the increased opportunities afforded to a person through cognitive or affective gene therapy preserve the identity of that same person. We aim to make *her* better off than *she* was before the intervention and thus provide her with the same opportunities as other people. By preserving her identity, the intervention would in fact be therapeutic. To insist on the utilitarian argument that it does not matter *who* has these opportunities, only *that* there are opportunities, fails to respect the distinctiveness of persons.[10] Beneficence and justice presuppose this idea of distinctiveness. While a principle of impersonal harm provides some support for the utilitarian argument for genetically improving mental functioning, a more persuasive version of this argument than what has been sketched here would have to be formulated for ignoring the distinctiveness of individual persons expressed in the more common egalitarian interpretation of beneficence and justice.

If the egalitarian view of benefit and opportunity is more persuasive than the utilitarian view, then there may be reasons for *not* using cognitive gene therapy on severely mentally impaired individuals. These reasons would be even stronger in the case of a moderate to moderately severe cognitive disability, as in Down syndrome. Why try to raise the level of cognitive and affective functioning and change the identity of persons if their mental capacities are sufficient for happy and fulfilling lives? It seems, that genetic intervention that improves one's mental functioning, preserves one's identity, and is genuinely therapeutic would be the type that *restores* individuals to normal functioning, not the type that significantly *raises* the mental functioning of moderately or severely mentally disabled individuals to a normal level.

Still, this point poses a challenge to the egalitarian idea of giving absolute priority to the worst off, which underscores its counterintuitive implications for cognitive gene therapy. Let us assume that an individual who has been cognitively impaired from birth is worse off in his life as a whole than one who has suddenly fallen below the baseline of adequate cognitive function due to a brain injury. If genetic intervention into the latter's brain will restore him to the baseline, and if the same sort of intervention does little to improve the condition of the former, then priority to the worse off individual can be overridden. This is because the benefit in being restored to the baseline of adequate mental functioning is more significant than the benefit in only marginally ameliorating the condition of the more severely affected individual.

The worst-off priority principle says that a smaller benefit to the worse off has more moral weight than a larger benefit to the better off.[11] But if the aim of any form of therapy is to raise or restore people to a decent minimum level of physical and mental functioning, then the significance of reaching that level for the better off may be enough for their claim to treatment to trump the claim of the worse off. It is morally preferable to benefit the better off and restore them to the decent minimum than to benefit others who are worse off if doing so only slightly improves their condition and fails to raise them to that level. Furthermore, suppose that the condition of the worse off could in fact be raised to the baseline of adequate mental functioning. Intuitively, this would make a strong case for giving priority to them. But if the improvement involved radical changes in the nature and content of their mental states, then they in fact would not be made better off, since they would not be the same persons after the intervention. This is quite unlike the case of restoring the better-off person to the baseline, since his mental states would effectively be re-connected as a result of the therapy, and his identity would be preserved. The coherence and justification of cognitive gene therapy hinges crucially on the preservation of personal identity and whether the purpose of therapy is restoring or raising people to a baseline of adequate mental functioning.

Conclusion

The safety of somatic-cell gene therapy and germ-line genetic intervention has yet to be established. Recently reported deaths in clinical trials involving gene therapy in the United States would suggest that the risk of harm may be considerable.[12] Indeed, many would hold that these deaths underscore that the moral issue of balancing benefits and harms looms larger than the metaphysical question of identity which I have explored here. This is especially significant in the case of germ-line intervention, since any adverse effects of a single intervention would be passed on to offspring and future generations of people, all of whom could be harmed by the defeat of their interest in having reasonably long and disease-free lives. The question of the trade-offs between the potential benefit and potential harm of all forms of genetic intervention to people will continue to figure prominently in philosophical and public debate about human genetics. But this debate cannot ignore the question of *who* stands to benefit or be harmed by genetic intervention, which underscores the importance of the influence of genetics on personal identity.

Notes

1   Antonio Damasio (1994) offers a sustained defense of the body's role in perception and self-consciousness in *Descartes' Error: Reason, Emotion, and the Human Brain*, New York, Grosset/Putnam, Ch.10, 'The Body-Minded Brain', and in *The Feeling of What Happens: Body and Emotion in the Making of Consciousness (1999)*, New York, Harcourt Brace.

2   Ibid., p.202 ff. Also, David Lewis, 'Survival and Identity', in A. O. Rorty, (ed.) (1976), *The Identities of Persons,* Berkeley, University of California Press, pp.17-40, Peter Unger (1990), *Identity, Consciousness, and Value,* New York, Oxford University Press, and Thomas Nagel (1985), *The View From Nowhere,* New York, Oxford University Press.

3   See, for example, Jeff McMahan, *The Ethics of Killing,* Oxford, Oxford University Press, 2002, Ch. 1, 'Personal Identity', and Ingmar Persson (1995), 'Genetic Therapy, Identity, and the Person-Regarding Reasons', *Bioethics* 9, pp.16-31. Cf. Eric Olson (1997), *The Human Animal: Personal Identity Without Psychology,* Oxford, Clarendon Press.

4   See especially Stephen Buckle (1988), who argues for the distinction between the potential to *become* and the potential to *produce* in 'Arguing from Potential', *Bioethics* vol. 2, p.227 ff. Also, Jonathan Glover (1977), *Causing Death and Saving Lives,* Harmondsworth, Penguin, p.128 ff. And John Harris (1998), *Clones, Genes, and Immortalit,* Oxford, Oxford University Press, p.8 ff.

5   See Joel Feinberg (1992), 'Wrongful Life and the Counterfactual Element in Harming', in *Freedom and Fulfillment,* Princeton, Princeton University Press, pp.3-36, David Heyd (1992), *Genethics: Moral Issues in the Creation of People,* Berkeley, University of California Press, Ch. 1, Harris, *Clones, Genes, and Immortality,* Ch. 4, and McMahan (1999), 'Wrongful Life: Paradoxes in the Morality of Causing People to Exist', in J. Coleman and C. Morris (eds), *Rational Commitment and Social Justice: Essays for Gregory Kavka,* Cambridge, Cambridge University Press, pp.208-247.

6   This is what Parfit calls the 'Full Comparative Requirement' in *Reasons and Persons,* p.488.

7   Among those who mistakenly call this 'therapy' are Leroy Walters and Julie Gage Palmer (1997), *The Ethics of Human Gene Therapy,* Oxford, Oxford University Press, Chs. 2 and 3, Persson (1995), 'Genetic Therapy, Identity, and the Person-Regarding Reasons', and Robert Elliott (1997), 'Genetic Therapy, Person-Regarding Reasons, and the Determination of Identity', *Bioethics* vol. 11, pp.151-160.

8   See Feinberg (1984), *Harm to Others,* New York, Oxford University Press.

9   McMahan (1996), 'Cognitive Disability, Misfortune, and Justice', *Philosophy & Public Affairs* vol. 25, pp.3-35, and Allen Buchanan (1996), 'Choosing Who Will Be Disabled: Genetic Intervention and the Morality of Inclusion', *Social Philosophy and Policy* vol. 13, pp.18-46.

10   John Rawls (1971), for one, criticizes utilitarianism for this reason in *A Theory of Justice,* Cambridge, MA, Belknap Harvard Press, p.27 ff.

11   Rawls, ibid., pp.1-27, 78-79, and 'Social Unity and Primary Goods', in B. Williams and A. Sen, (eds) (1982), *Utilitarianism and Beyond,* Cambridge, Cambridge University Press, pp.162-163. Also Nagel (1991), *Equality and Partiality,* Oxford, Oxford University Press, 1991, Larry Temkin (1993), *Inequality,* Oxford, Oxford University Press, and Parfit (1995), 'Equality or Priority?', Lindley Lecture, Lawrence, KS, University of Kansas Press.

12   In an article in the *New York Times,* it was claimed that Jesse Gelsinger, who suffered from a mild form of omithine transcarbamylase (OTC) deficiency, a disorder in which the liver cannot process ammonia, a toxic breakdown product of food, died as a result of gene therapy using a viral vector at the University of Pennsylvania. See 'Youth's Death Jars Gene-Therapy Field', *New York Times,* January 21, 2000. Also, on May 3, 2000 it was reported that a patient died after receiving gene therapy involving vascular endothelial growth factor (VEGF) at St. Elizabeth's Hospital in Boston. 'A Second Death Linked to Gene Therapy', *New York Times,* May 4, 2000.

References

Austin, J. (1989), *Human Embryos: The Debate on Assisted Reproduction,* Oxford, Oxford University Press, p.17.

Buchanan, A. (1996), 'Choosing Who Will Be Disabled: Genetic Intervention and the Morality of Inclusion', *Social Philosophy and Policy* vol. 13, pp.18-46.

Buckle, S. (1988), 'Arguing from Potential', *Bioethics* vol. 2, pp.224-233.

Cavazzana-Calvo, M. et al. (2000), 'Gene Therapy of Human Severe Combined Immunodeficiency (SCID)—X1 Disease', *Science* vol. 288, pp.669-672.

Coleman, J. and Morris, C. (1999), *Rational Commitment and Social Justice: Essays for Greogry Kavka*, Cambridge, Cambridge University Press.

Damasio, A. (1994), *Descartes' Error: Reason, Emotion, and the Human Brain*, New York, Grosset/Putnam.

Damasio, A. (1999), *The Feeling of What Happens: Body and Emotion in the Making of Consciousness*, New York, Harcourt Brace.

Elliott, R. (1997), 'Genetic Therapy, Person-Regarding Reasons, and the Determination of Identity', *Bioethics* vol. 11, pp.151-160.

Feinberg, J. (1984), *Harm to Others*, New York, Oxford University Press.

Feinberg, J. (1992), 'Wrongful Life and the Counterfactual Element in Harming', in *Freedom and Fulfillment*, Princeton, Princeton University Press, pp.3-36.

Glover, J. (1977), *Causing Death and Saving Lives*, Harmondsworth, Penguin.

Harris, J. (1998), *Clones, Genes, and Immortaltiy*, Oxford, Oxford University Press.

Heyd, D. (1992), *Genethics: Moral Issues in the Creation of People*, Berkeley, University of California Press.

Lewis, D. (1976), 'Survival and Identity', in Rorty, *The Identities of Persons*, pp.17-40.

McMahan, J. (1999), 'Wrongful Life: Paradoxes in the Morality of Causing People to Exist', in Coleman and Morris, pp.208-247.

McMahan, J. (2002), *The Ethics of Killing*, Oxford, Oxford University Press.

Nagel, T. (1985), *The View From Nowhere*, New York, Oxford University Press.

Nagel, T. (1991), *Equality and Partiality*, Oxford, Oxford University Press.

Olson, E. (1997), *The Human Animal: Personal Identity Without Psychology*, Oxford, Clarendon Press.

Parfit, D. (1976), 'Lewis, Perry, and What Matters', in A. O. Rorty, (ed.), *The Identities of Persons,* Berkeley, University of California Press, p.103, n.10.

Parfit, D. (1984), *Reasons and Persons*, Oxford, Clarendon Press, p.202.

Parfit, D. (1995), 'Equality or Priority?', Lindley Lecture, Lawrence, KS, University of Kansas Press.

Persson, I. (1995), 'Genetic Therapy, Identity, and the Person-Regarding Reasons', *Bioethics* vol. 9, pp.16-31.

Rawls, J. (1971), *A Theory of Justice*, Cambridge, MA, Belknap Harvard Press.

Rawls, J. (1982), 'Social Unity and Primary Goods', in Williams and Sen, pp.162-182.

Rorty, A. (ed.) (1976), *The Identities of Persons*, Berkeley, University of California Press.

Silver, L. (1997), *Remaking Eden,* New York, Avon Books, p.64.

Tang, Y.-P. et al. (1999), 'Genetic Enhancement of Learning and Memory in Mice', *Science* vol. 286, pp.63-69.

Temkin, L. (1993), *Inequality*, Oxford, Oxford University Press.

Walters, L. and Palmer, J. (1997), *The Ethics of Human Gene Therapy*, New York, Oxford University Press.

Williams, B. and Sen, A. (1982), *Utilitarianism and Beyond*, Cambridge, Cambridge University Press.

Wolfe, A.P. and Matzke, M.A. (1999), 'Epigenetics: Regulation Through Repression', *Science* vol. 286, p.481-486.

PART 2

Genetics, Determinism and Personal Identity

Chapter 8

Genetic Reductionism and the Concepts of Health and Disease

Tom Buller

The previous chapter has raised the question of whether genetic intervention for medical reasons affects a person's (or an embryo's) continuing identity, and in this chapter, I pursue some assumptions that prompt people to ask this question. So are health and disease really completely genetically determined? It seems that many, including many distinguished authorities, take for granted some form of genetic reductionism, for example, as John Watson has put the matter, 'our fate is in our genes', and are increasingly likely to understand health and disease in genetic terms. My focus in this chapter, however, is not directly on the question of whether health and disease are completely genetically determined (in fact, I think this claim is false) but on whether genetic reductionism is reshaping the way in which think about health and disease. Specifically, I consider whether recent developments in genetics will lead us to revise or even possibly replace our existing theory of health and disease with a new genetic one.

In a recent article in *TIME* about the successful near-completion of the Human Genome Project (HGP), the authors wrote:

> Armed with the new genetic code, scientists can now start teasing out the secrets of human health and disease at the molecular level–secrets that will lead at the very least to a revolution in diagnosing and treating everything from Alzheimer's to heart disease to cancer, and more. In a matter of decades, the world of medicine will be utterly transformed, and history books will mark this week as the ceremonial start of the genomic era. (Golden and Lemonick, 2000)

In this chapter I want to explore one aspect of this predicted revolution, namely the effect that our greater understanding of the humane genome and molecular genetics will have on our present concepts of health and disease. In particular, I am interested in the view that a person's health status is genetically determined and that underlies the sentiments expressed above. This view is often referred to as 'genetic reductionism'. My intention in this paper is not to defend genetic reductionism but to discuss its claims and merits, and to consider whether genetic reductionism presents a new theory of health and disease that will compete with, and possible replace our present theory.

Genetic reductionism as genetic determinism

When genetic reductionism is discussed, it is generally understood in causal terms as the thesis that genes are responsible for determining health and disease. More precisely, genetic reductionism can be understood in terms of the following claims: firstly, further research will continue to reveal that many diseases have a genetic aetiology; and secondly, that a person's future health is causally dependent, in considerable part, on the presence or absence of predisposing disease traits in the person's genetic make-up. To put the point in epistemic terms, once we have all the necessary genetic information we will be able to predict a person's future health. To some extent these claims might appear uncontroversial for there is good evidence to suggest that genetics (biology) does play an important role in health and disease; however, the version of genetic reductionism that seems to underlie the sentiments above is rather more far-reaching, and thus more controversial, since it appears to claim that many (if not most) diseases are genetic, and that genetics plays the *central* role in determining a person's health. This more radical version of genetic reductionism has been termed 'genetic imperialism' (Juengst, 2000).

Perhaps not surprisingly, genetic imperialism has few supporters. For the following reasons it is argued that although genes play some role in determining a person's health, genetic imperialism grossly overstates their causal importance. To begin with, although one can readily grant that genetics plays some role in the development of disease and a person's health, most (if not all) diseases are multifactoral - there are other factors in addition to a person's genetics that are relevant to the onset of disease, for example, the person's socio-economic status and occupation, the environment in which he or she lives, and the lifestyle that is followed. Thus a knowledge of the genetic factors will not enable us to predict a person's health status. As Robert Proctor says:

> Genetics is not going to explain the fact that asbestos miners have higher mesothelioma rates than people who work in air-conditioned offices, nor will it explain the fact that people who live in homes with radon seepage are more likely to contract cancer. (1992, p.344)

Another reason for rejecting genetic imperialism is that the possession of a genetic trait should be regarded as neither necessary nor sufficient for developing a particular disease. To take breast cancer as an example: a person may develop the disease even though he or she lacks both of the genetic traits for familial breast cancer (BRCA1/BRCA2), and a person may not develop the disease even though she does, in fact, possess these traits.

A final reason to be skeptical of genetic imperialism is that the majority of diseases are polygenic rather than single-gene disorders, and the inherited risk of developing a disease is produced not by the effects of a single gene mutation but by 'a much larger number of susceptibility and protective genes each contributing small effects' (Marteau and Richards, 1999). As Eric Juengst says:

As medicine re-learns human physiology from the genome up, genetic multi-potency is likely to become the norm rather than the exception: every genotypic change probably has multiple phenotypic effects, just as any particular effect is likely to have multiple genotypic causes. (Op. cit. p.125)

In other words, the causal connections that underlie genetic imperialism are far more complicated than genetic imperialism suggests, and it is highly unlikely that we will find the one-to-one match-ups between the manifestation of a disease and a single gene mutation.

Two theories of health and disease

On the basis of the above it would appear that genetic reductionism should be abandoned, and that we should, perhaps, be rather more modest in the claims we make about the impact of the completion of the Human Genome Project and other developments. This clearly would be the appropriate conclusion to draw if the causal view of genetic imperialism were the only possible version of genetic reductionism; one can, however, understand genetic reductionism in other ways. One alternative to genetic imperialism is to regard genetic reductionism as primarily a methodological approach rather than as a substantive theory. As Jonathan Kaplan claims, although few might support genetic reductionism as a theory, many of those who profess their opposition to genetic determinism would agree with the methodological perspective that 'the genetic is the natural place to look when attempting to explain, predict, and control traits with even partial genetic etiologies' (Kaplan, 2000, p.12).

Another possible alternative is to consider genetic reductionism not as a causal theory but in the more orthodox sense of reductionism as pertaining to the relationship between properties, concepts and theories. In general terms, a reductionist account claims that there is one set of properties, concepts, or explanations where previously we thought there were two, for example, the reduction of heat to molecular energy, or more controversially, the reduction of mental states to neurochemical brain states. To talk of one thing being reduced to another is to say that the reduced property *just is* the reducing one, for example, temperature is now understood to be nothing but mean molecular energy (Heil, 1998). When an existing theory is challenged by a new theory with greater explanatory success or greater generality (Charles and Lennon, 1992, p.5), the existing theory can survive if it can be shown that there are law-like connections that relate the concepts and properties of the existing theory to those of the new. If the properties and concepts of the existing theory and the new cannot be related in this way, then the likely outcome is that the existing theory will be replaced; (successful) reduction can, therefore, be seen as a way of preserving the autonomy of the reduced theory.

In the present context, genetic reductionism can be understood, therefore, in terms of the revision or possible replacement of our existing theory of health and disease by a new genetic theory of health and disease. What are the existing and new theories? Broadly speaking, our existing theory of health and disease can be understood in terms of the 'three F's': the physiological; the functional; and the phenomenological. When we say that a person has a disease, for example, colon cancer or Alzheimer's Dementia, we understand the person to be no longer able to function to the same degree as before the onset of the disease, and that, other things being equal, the person is in pain or suffering; furthermore, we expect that we will be able to identify some physiological basis for this loss of function and the direct or indirect pain and suffering. If none of these conditions are met then we would be led to question the conclusion that the person has a disease.

Another aspect that marks our traditional concept of disease, and those of diagnosis, symptom, and treatment is that the three conditions have to be *presently* met; that is to say, we tend not to think of a person as *having* colon cancer if the person does not presently have the disease but will develop it at some time in the future; in other words, we reject, either implicitly or explicitly, the notion that having a predisposition for a disease is the same as actually having the disease - potentiality is not actuality (Ommen et al., 1999).

This existing view of health and disease is being challenged by the recent developments in genetics, however. As a result of our successful mapping and sequencing of the human genome, we have seen a marked increase in the number of diseases that are recognized as having major genetic components. Furthermore, as our knowledge and ability regarding genetic testing, screening, and therapy increases, there is evidence to suggest that we are beginning to think of health and disease in terms of the presence or absence of genetic traits, rather than in terms of physiology, function and phenomenology. As evidence that we have already begun to shift our allegiance from the existing theory of disease to the new, one can point to the way in which we now think of genetic testing as 'diagnostic;', and describe a disease at the stage before symptoms develop as 'presymptomatic' i.e. present rather than absent (Juengst, op. cit., p.129). Relatedly, we talk of the replacement of defective genes by non-defective ones as 'gene therapy', even though what is being attempted is not something that would be thought of as therapeutic on our existing theory, since gene therapy seeks to prevent the development of a disease rather than to cure or heal the person. Furthermore, if we consider the case of prenatal testing by amniocentesis for conditions such as Down's Syndrome, there is a tendency to view a positive test result (one revealing the presence of *Trisomy 21*) as showing that the foetus *has* Down's, even though none of the functional, physical or phenomenological elements that are typically associated with Down's are yet present, and nor can the degree to which the condition manifests itself be determined at that time. The same type of consideration seems to be behind other cases where a positive genetic test reveals that the person carries the disease gene; for example, the decision by some women with a familial history of breast cancer to have both breasts and ovaries removed prophylactically. And a similar conception seems to be shared by those who argue that insurance companies should have access to the genetic information of someone seeking insurance. Presumably, someone who is known to be predisposed to develop a disease would be viewed differently from a person with no such predisposition, and this information would be relevant to the insurance company in its decision to insure the person at the present time. All of these examples suggest that the new theory of health and disease blurs the distinction between present and future health.

In light of the objections to genetic imperialism above regarding the importance of environmental causes, it might be objected that we should not think that being predisposed to develop a disease is the same as having the disease, for if the presence or absence of genetic traits does not meaningfully determine a person's future health, then we are simply mistaken to think of genetic tests as diagnostic or the disease at this early state as present but presymptomatic. It is in these terms that one can respond to the claims of insurance companies mentioned above. However, it is important to notice that this objection is itself dependant on the existing theoretical conception of health and disease whereby health is conceived of in terms of physiological, functional and phenomenological elements. The success of the argument that genetic traits do not equal having the disease rests on the assumption that a person has a disease only if the physical, functional, and phenomenological elements are present. However, this is the very notion being questioned since the genetic theory of disease does not see disease in these terms. At present we tend not to think that a person who is found to have the genetic traits for heritable breast cancer *has* the disease because we think that in order for the person to actually have the disease the physical, functional and phenomenological elements must be present. As our knowledge of genetics and our predictions of disease improve, however, it is possible that we could come to regard the possession of the traits as what it means to have the disease; in other words, we would redefine the concept of disease.

It needs to be said that there may be independent reasons for not redefining disease in this way. In particular, there is legitimate concern about the use and misuse of genetic information as a result of the Human Genome Project. We may want to resist redefining the concept of disease on the grounds that to do so would have adverse social consequences.[1] If we come to regard the possession of a disease treat as equivalent to having the disease and allow insurance companies and other institutions to have this information, then there is good reason to suppose that those who have the disease treat will be adversely affected.

The success of a theory depends in considerable part on its explanatory success, and the extent to which the theory appears to be 'closer to a characterization of the basic or real causal mechanisms' (Charles and Lennon, op. cit., p.5). On the basis of the objections to genetic imperialism above we might be led to conclude that, since the genetic theory of disease incorrectly characterizes the causal elements, it is no better than or present theory of health and disease. Whether or not we will be led to this conclusion depends on what we imagine future genetic research to reveal. If we believe that future research will, in fact, reveal the influence of genes to be much greater than presently realized, then the new genetic theory of disease may be seen to have the characterization correct; on the other hand, if we believe that the future gains of research will confirm the limited role that genes play, then we may continue to regard the genetic theory of disease as providing at best but one part of the overall picture.

The subjectivity and normativity of health

One way in which our old theory of health and disease could resist replacement by the new genetic theory is if we could find the appropriate match-ups between the properties and concepts in our old theory with those of the new, and thereby reduce the old theory to the new. This is in part an empirical question about the possibility of discovering the generality of genetics and the extent to which we can incorporate the physiological, functional and phenomenological elements into our genetic and biological theories, finding the appropriate match-ups between these concepts and elements in the reducing genetic theory. Perhaps we will discover that a person's tolerance for pain and suffering has a genetic basis, or we will be able to more accurately match up genotypic causes with phenotypic effects. The more we discover that our present concepts of health and disease are mirrored in genetics, the greater the likelihood of reduction. Another way one might challenge the possibility of a successful reduction of our existing theory of health and disease to the genetic theory is by pointing to elements in our existing theory that it is claimed cannot be reduced.

There is good reason, perhaps, to think that we will not be able to find the appropriate match-ups. There are two elements that are often regarded as stumbling blocks to reductionism in other discussions, namely subjectivity and normativity. The phenomenological aspect of disease, the experience of health or sickness, plays a central role in our existing theory of health and disease. This element is of considerable importance because first-person accounts of illness help us to understand what it means to have a disease, and are of considerable use to others who are ill and those responsible for treating them.[2] It is difficult to see, however, how we would be able to include this element if we conceive of disease in mostly genetic terms, for it is difficult to see how the notion of subjectivity can be included in the objective, non-perspectival world of genetics and biology in which the experiences of health and disease are absent. There seems to be no place for the phenomenological at the physical, genetic level, and so it is difficult to see how this element could be reduced.

A second property that resists reduction is normativity. If we consider on what basis we judge one state of health to be worse than another, for example, having AIDS as opposed to not having it, it seems clear that it is only if the disease manifests itself that we are able to distinguish these two states evaluatively. If we consider the two states simply in terms of their genetic characteristics and in isolation from their predicted physical, functional and phenomenological qualities, there does not seem to be any standard that we could use to say that one state is any better or worse than the other; for at this level states can be differentiated only in terms of their biological composition. In other words, until and unless the disease manifests itself, we would have no justification or basis for thinking that one biological state is worse than another. One objection to this might be to claim that there are teleological considerations that apply 'all the way down' - we can describe a genetic trait as abnormal because it is unusual and because we have reason to believe it will impair the functioning of the system. However, since it is possible for there to be genetic abnormalities that do not negatively affect a person's health, it is not clear that these teleological considerations correspond with our notions of health and disease.

It is difficult to predict the effect that the recent developments will have on our existing theory of health and disease, and it is possible that as advances in genetics continue our existing theory of health and disease will remain unscathed. I hope this chapter has shown, however, that there is reason to believe that the developments in genetics are challenging our existing theory to the degree to which either our existing theory will be subsumed under the new theory, or it will be replaced. While these complex issues remain unresolved, I hope to have shown how much impact the Human Genome Project has had on our existing concepts of health and disease, and that this will prompt further discussion about the claims of genetic reductionism.

Notes

1   For example, in addition to the works by Proctor, Marteau and Richards, Juengst and Kaplan cited above, Daniel Kevles and Leroy Hood (eds) (1993), *The Code of Codes: Scientific and Social Issues in the Human Genome Project*, Harvard, Harvard University Press, pp.177-328.

2   See for example, Holly F. Matthews, Donald R. Lannin, and James P. Mitchell, 'Coming to Terms with Advanced Breast Cancer: Black Women's Narratives from Eastern North Carolina', in Gail E. Henderson, Nancy M. P. King, Ronald P. Straus, Sue E. Estroff, and Larry Churchill (eds) (1997), *The Social Medicine Reader*, Duke University Press, p.43-61.

References

Charles, D. and Lennon, K. (1992), *Reduction, Explanation, and Realism*, (eds), Oxford, Clarendon Press, p.5.

Golden, F. and Lemonick, M.D. 'The Quest is Over', *TIME* July 3, 2000.

Heil, J. (1998), *Philosophy of Mind: A Contemporary Introduction*, London, Routledge, p.169.

Juengst, E. (2000), 'Concepts of Disease After The Human Genome Project', in *Ethical Issues in Health Care on the Frontiers of the Twenty-First Century*, S. Wear, J.J. Bono, G. Logue and A. McEvoy, Dordrecht, Holland, Kluwer (eds), pp.125-152.

Kaplan, J.M. (2000), *The Limits and Lies of Human Genetic Research: Dangers for Social Policy*, London, Routledge, p.12.

Marteau, T. and Richards, M. (eds) (1999), *The Troubled Helix: Social and Psychological Implications of the New Genetics*, Cambridge, Cambridge University Press, p.xvii.

Proctor, R.N. (1992), 'Resisting Reductionism from the Human Genome Project', in *Gene Mapping: A Guide to Law and Ethics*, Annas, G. and Elias, S. (eds), Oxford, Oxford University Press, reprinted in Gregory E. Pence (1998), *Classic Works in Medical Ethics*, McGraw-Hill, pp.341-349, 344.

Van Ommen, G.B., Baker, E., and den Dunnen, J.T. (1999), 'The Human Genome Project and the Future of Diagnostics, Treatment, and Prevention', *The Lancet*, vol.354 (suppl. 1) pp.5-10.

Chapter 9

From Catch-Phrase to Catechism: the Central Dogma in Molecular Biology[1]

Robyn Bluhm

Since 1953, when James Watson and Francis Crick first determined the structure of the DNA molecule, scientists have learned a great deal about the human genome and its role in human development. Much of this progress has been made possible by the adoption of a particular conception of our genetic machinery, known as the 'central dogma'. The central dogma states that information flows in one direction only: from Dioxi-ribonucleic-acid, to ribonucleic-acid, to protein. The central dogma, while useful in the laboratory, does not provide an adequate explanation of the role of the genes in real-life development. DNA provides a blueprint from which living creatures are constructed; however, communication between the molecules involved in that construction resembles a richly interconnected network, rather than the linear chain of command implied by the central dogma.

In this chapter, I argue that the simplified view of development implied by the central dogma is not limited to the laboratory. It is also reflected in the way that genetic research is treated in the media, and ultimately affects our understanding of our bodies and of our selves. But just as the central dogma fails to do complete justice to the molecular level, the genetic determinism it inspires does not adequately reflect what it means to be a human being. I will show that the modern version of the central dogma was influenced by social factors, and argue that it, in turn, has come to influence our culture's understanding of genetics and development. There is no doubt that genetic research will affect all of us – what must be ensured is that we have the conceptual resources to adequately assess its impact. We need a richer understanding of molecular interactions than the central dogma can provide.

Every day, it seems, we hear of new progress in genetic research. The Human Genome Project is near completion, and genes are being discovered that influence our chances of having various kinds of cancer, a heart attack or Alzheimer's disease. While the previous chapter has focussed on the issue of health and disease, genetic explanations are not limited to health issues. Personality traits and social behaviors are often explained with reference to our genes.[2] Dorothy Nelkin cites articles in which a genetic basis is suggested for 'shyness, directional ability, aggressive personality, exhibitionism, homosexuality, dyslexia, job success, political leanings, religiosity, infidelity, intelligence, social potency and zest for life' (Nelkin, 1995, p.27). While we can also explain these characteristics in psychological or sociological terms we tend to think of genetic differences as being somehow more fundamental. Abby Lippman calls the process by which we come to focus on genetic explanation 'geneticization'. In this process, 'differences between individuals are reduced to their DNA codes, with most disorders, behaviors and physiological variations defined, at least in part, as genetic in origin...Through this process, human biology is incorrectly equated with human genetics, implying that the latter acts alone to make us each the organism she or he is' (1991, p.19).

According to Nelkin and Lindee (1995), ours is a culture fascinated by the gene. It is popular to imagine individual and social characteristics as explicable by 'something in the genes'. Certainly the media coverage of molecular research is generally favorable; it suggests that once we understand how our genes work, and what happens when they go wrong, we will be able to prevent or cure disease, eradicate birth defects, and treat complex behavioral disorders such as alcoholism and schizophrenia. Certainly, a better understanding of genetics will create new options for medical diagnosis and treatment. But we need to understand that genetic explanations, on their own, are rarely enough.

The term 'central dogma' was introduced by Francis Crick in 1957. At that time, very little was known about the process by which proteins were synthesized, and Crick was simply speculating on the process by which sequence information contained in a molecule of DNA might be transferred to a protein. In a paper published the following year, Crick describes two general principles: the sequence hypothesis and the central dogma. Both principles, according to Crick, are of a 'speculative nature' (Crick, 1958, p.152), and he notes that '[t]he direct evidence for both of them is negligible' (ibid.). However, he suggests that the use of these principles makes it easier to think about the complex process of protein synthesis.

The sequence hypothesis suggests that the order of the nucleic acids in a strand of DNA codes for the specific sequence of amino acids to be found in a protein. The central dogma 'states that once "information" has passed into protein *it cannot get out again*' (ibid., p.153). By 'information', Crick meant simply 'the *precise* determination of sequence, either of bases in the nucleic acid or of amino acid residues in the protein' (ibid.). Sarkar (1998) notes that this formulation of the central dogma is in negative terms, as it forbids the flow of information from protein to protein, protein to RNA, or protein to DNA. Again, however, in this original paper, Crick recognizes that proof for either hypothesis is 'completely lacking' (Crick, p.161). He concludes with the suggestion that 'protein synthesis is a central problem for the whole of biology and that it is *in all probability* closely related to gene action' (ibid., p.160, italics mine).

Over the next couple of decades, new techniques in molecular biology provided experimental support for both principles. By the mid 1960s, scientists understood the genetic code relating the sequence of a gene to that of the protein for which it codes. Further research also clarified the mechanisms by which information could be transferred according to the central dogma. Over time, however, the sequence hypothesis became enveloped into the central dogma, and the central dogma itself began to be more rigidly interpreted. By 1965, the central dogma was described as the claim that there is a linear, unidirectional flow of information from DNA to RNA to protein (e.g. Watson, 1965).

In this restatement of the dogma, the focus shifts from the proteins being synthesized to the genes carrying the hereditary information governing this synthesis. The reasons for this change, however, can only be understood in the context of the history of molecular biology. This emphasis on the gene reflects a tendency among biologists, existing well before Crick's formulation of the central dogma, to adopt a reductive approach to inherited characteristics. Even before the 1953 discovery, by Watson and Crick, of the structure of the DNA molecule, the gene was viewed as the fundamental source of all the traits possessed by an organism.

It is important to realize that research into the mechanisms of heredity during the early 20th century took place along side the eugenics movement (described in Kay, 1993, Ch.1; Hubbard and Wald 1997, Ch.2). This movement advocated selective breeding a way to improve the human race. Eugenicists envisioned a sort of artificial selection, which would ensure that only the fittest, most desirable genes survived.

Of course eugenics was also a form of genetic determinism, as it reduced differences between individuals to differences between individual genomes. Evelyn Fox Keller writes of 'the discourse of gene action', the way of thinking that views genes as the *cause* of biological traits and sees the goal of biology as the understanding of how genes act. She shows that this discourse arises because of the gradual separation, in the early part of the 20th century of embryology (viewed as the study of development from a single fertilized egg to a mature organism) and genetics (which was concerned with 'tracking the transmission of differences among existing organisms') (1995, p.6). This separation also resulted in a change in the use of the term 'heredity' – which once described both the 'transmission of potentialities during reproduction *and* [the] development of these potentialities into specific adult characteristics' (Allen, 1958, quoted in Keller, 1995, p.4) – to refer solely to transmission. Thus, heredity became associated with genetics.

At this time, scientists were still uncertain as to the nature of the gene. Early geneticists used the term 'gene' in a purely functional sense: it referred to the thing or substance that was responsible for passing inherited traits from parent to offspring. (Used in this sense, a gene could transmit a simple characteristic, such as those studied by Mendel, or a complex one, like intelligence.) Molecular geneticists used the techniques of physics and chemistry to try to determine the structure of the gene, and their research was influenced by the geneticists' definition. The gene was thought to be unchanging, and capable of self-replication. These two characteristics ensured that a new generation resembled its parents.

In the lab, these biases were reflected in the kinds of research being conducted. The 'protein paradigm' (described in Kay, 1993, and Olby, 1975) of the 1930's and 40's concentrated on the parallels between the (as yet unidentified) genetic material and autocatalytic enzymes. These enzymes, as their name suggests, were able to catalyze their own synthesis, so that, in a sense, they brought themselves into being. The gene was conceptualized as a protein with similar powers; it contained both the information specifying the traits to be inherited, and instructions for the use of that information.

While proteins were still the topic of much research during the 1940s, it became increasingly clear that nucleic acids played an important role in heredity. Still, the change was slow. Even though published evidence existed as early as 1944 that DNA, not proteins, was responsible for transmitting inherited characteristics, the focus of research shifted only gradually from proteins to nucleic acids. In his autobiography, Watson notes that when he arrived in Cambridge in 1951, there were still 'scientists who thought that the evidence favoring DNA was inconclusive and preferred to think that genes were protein molecules' (p.18).

The 1953 discovery of the structure of DNA, with its implications for 'a possible copying mechanism for the genetic material' (Watson and Crick, 1953 p.4356) provided a decisive victory for scientists engaged in nucleic acid research. It also strengthened the case for genetic determinism. As Crick notes, 'the most significant thing about proteins is that they can do almost anything' (1958, p.138), from providing structural support to a cell to catalyzing almost all of the chemical reactions that occur in it. By contrast, it seemed that 'the main function of the genetic material is to control (not necessarily directly) the synthesis of proteins' (ibid.). Unlike proteins, which are complex, varied and messy, DNA appears pristine and unchanging – well suited to the task of transmitting immutable characteristics from generation to generation.

The equation of heredity with transmission and the concept of the gene as self-replicating and unchanging influenced genetic research during the 1950s and 60s, and also contributed to the shift in interpretation of the central dogma. The work of Watson and Crick 'began as a narrowly defined and proper theory and paradigm of the gene, [but] has mistakenly evolved into a theory and a paradigm of life: That is, into a revived and thoroughly molecular form of genetic determinism' (Strohman, 1997, p.194).

As genetics turned into molecular biology, and became more and more successful at solving the problem of transmission, it began to encroach on the territory of embryologists as well. The language of geneticists and molecular biologists began to be used to describe development. Rather than a complex process of interaction between many kinds of molecules, development began to be described as the unfolding of a pre-existing program located, of course, in the sequence of base pairs in the DNA. In 1993, James Watson claimed that 'developmental biologists, who do not think in terms of DNA, are relics of the past with little likelihood to influence the future' (p.313).

This view of development assumes that the genome contains all of the information necessary for the development of the organism. It also downplays the differences between the mechanisms involved in the synthesis of DNA and that of proteins. The first process, known as replication, copies the entire genome and passes it to a new generation of cells. Gene expression involves only a part of the genome, and is the process by which proteins are synthesized. Replication underlies heredity in the narrow sense of passing genetic material to a new generation. Gene expression is the process by which this genetic information is used during the development of an organism or cell. The central dogma, though originally developed to explain protein synthesis (and therefore gene expression) also touches on the process of replication since it allows information to pass from one strand of DNA to a new strand. Both gene expression and replication are much more complex than the central dogma would suggest.[3]

DNA replication occurs in two instances. In the first case, the DNA is passed from one generation of organisms to the next: animals receive half of their DNA from each parent, and while each parent passes on only half of his or her DNA to the offspring, the genes are largely unchanged.[4] DNA is also inherited, in a sense, in the process of somatic cell division. In this case, the DNA of a single cell is replicated, and a copy is passed to each of two daughter cells. In both kinds of heredity, information passes from protein to DNA. Contrary to the initial hypothesis of the gene as an autocatalytic agent, it turns out that the replication of DNA relies on a host of enzymes: some of these are even responsible for correcting the sequence information in the DNA if an error is made in replication. Despite the claims of the central dogma, the structure of a DNA molecule depends on information from various proteins.

The main focus of the central dogma, however, is on gene expression. Protein synthesis underlies the process of growth and development, and this synthesis relies on the sequence information contained in an organism's genome. However, the central dogma implies that the gene is the primary agent in development. This is the molecular version of genetic determinism, of the view that 'it's all in our genes'.

In reality, this is far from the case. The cytoplasm of a fertilized egg contains genes and proteins that are not part of the new organism's own genome, but are contributed by the mother. During the first few divisions of the zygote these maternal contributions are not shared equally between the daughter cells, so that the cytoplasm of each of these cells is not the same. This is the beginning of the process of differentiation; the amount and kinds of chemicals in the cytoplasm of each cell influences *which* genes are expressed in protein synthesis, and how much protein is synthesized. As the embryonic development continues, the kinds of proteins expressed in a cell affect the further development of the cell and of neighboring cells, as well. These processes determine whether a cell will become part of the liver, or the heart, and which part of the heart or the liver it will become. Most important, the differentiation of a cell also affects its DNA: as a cell differentiates, a variety of proteins contribute to the 'silencing' of portions of the genome: the structure of the DNA molecule is changed so that some genes cannot be expressed (e.g. Beato, 1996; Carrington and Jones, 1996). As the cell divides, the change in DNA structure is inherited by the next cell generation (Loo and Rine, 1995), even if the proteins required for the initial silencing are not present in the cell at the time. It is not merely the sequence of DNA that is inherited by the daughter cells, it is also the molecule's higher-order shape. This shape is determined by the DNA's environment, and cannot be derived solely from the sequence.

Collectively, the mechanisms that influence gene expression are described as 'epigenetic networks'. Whereas the central dogma describes a linear flow of information, epigenetic mechanisms are more complex, and most likely non-linear

(Strohman, 1997). They are also influenced by signals from the environment, which is why the lifestyle choices made by someone with a genetic tendency to heart disease, or to a specific kind of cancer, can make such a difference – at a molecular level – to whether they develop the disease. Diet, exercise and occupation can all affect the intracellular environment in which gene expression takes place. The central dogma does not recognize any level but the molecular; it is able to account for the chemical results of human choices, but has no way of explaining the choices themselves. For that, we need a theoretical framework that can account for relationships between different levels of organization.

Richard Lewontin is one scientist who works within this kind of framework. He claims that development cannot be understood unless we recognize that it is a dialectical process. Only then can we appreciate the relationship between genes and organism, knowing that 'one thing cannot exist without the other, that one acquires its properties from its relation to the other, that the properties of both evolve as a consequence of their interpenetration' (Levins and Lewontin, 1985, p.3). Most scientific work proceeds reductively; it breaks complex wholes into their component parts, and explains the behavior of the whole as the product of the behavior of isolated parts. By contrast, a dialectical view recognizes that the relationship between parts and whole is complex. 'It is not that the whole is more than the sum of its parts. It is that the properties of the parts cannot be understood except in their context in the whole' (Lewontin, 1992, p.96). It makes no sense, then, to talk about 'gene action' as if that action were somehow separate from the organism of which those genes are a part.

Why, then, is genetic determinism so compelling? Lewontin points out that scientists are often 'devoted to the ideology of simple unitary causes' (ibid., p.51). In this, however, scientists are no different from the rest of us. And, of course, this ideology also implies that there are simple unitary solutions, that '[i]f only we could find those genes that underlie alcoholism or those that have gone awry when we get cancer, then our problems will be over' (ibid., p.46).

In fact, there are rarely simple solutions to genetic questions. Strohman estimates that only 2 per cent of diseases can be truly be considered 'real, genetic diseases' (1997, p.199). Other diseases may have a genetic component, it is true. Some people carry genes that predispose them to develop heart disease, for example. However, this does not mean that these genes *cause* the disease in any straightforward sense. It can just as truthfully be claimed that the cause was exposure to environmental toxins, lack of exercise or a diet too high in saturated fat. The difference in the two kinds of explanation is that, if we see the cause as genetic then we tend to feel that there is nothing we can do about our fate. If we claim that the cause is among the other factors, then our health becomes something that is, at least partly, under our control.

The importance of this way of thinking becomes even more evident when we analyze sociobiological theories. Sociobiologists describe complex behaviors and social structures in the language of genetic determinism. And, again, the reduction of (for example) gender relations, class structures and even the dynamics of the free market to genetic drives implies that none of these can be changed.

Of course, one does not have to be a sociobiologist to believe in the necessity of our political and economic structures. Like genes, these forces are often described as having a life of their own. Similarly, arguments against genetic determinism often parallel those of political theorists. John Ralston Saul suggests that, as a civilization, we have become addicted to 'large illusions, to the pursuit of all-inclusive truths' (1995, p.19). Genetic determinism is just as much an ideology as Marxism or Fascism. All of these rigid conceptual frameworks lead us to ask 'the great inapplicable questions: What is civilization? What is man?' (ibid., p.32). In addition, they force us to answer these questions in the terms of that ideology.

Like Lippman's concept of geneticization, these frameworks gradually transform the way we see the world until it is difficult for us to conceive of a world that does not conform to this ideological framework. The belief that we are, ultimately, our genes is another of Saul's 'large illusions' and is just as dangerous as any political determinism.

Notes

1   I would like to thank both the Department of Philosophy and the Graduate Students' Association at McMaster University, Hamilton, Ontario, Canada, for their generous support during the writing of this paper.
2   The field of sociobiology, strictly speaking, involves the study of the biological bases of social behavior. In practice, however, this often translates to genetic explanations (see, for example, Wilson, 1975).
3   Though, as Kuhn's theory predicts, it was the paradigm of the central dogma that led scientists to discover its own weaknesses.
4   Discounting, for now, mitochondrial DNA, which is inherited solely from the mother.

References

Allen, G. (1986), 'T.H. Morgan and the Split Between Embryology and Genetics, 1910-1926', in T.J. Horder, I.A. Witowski and C.C. Wylie (eds), *A History of Embryology*. Cambridge, Cambridge University Press, pp.151-168.

Beato, M. (1996), 'Chromatin Structure and the Regulation of Gene Expression: Remodeling at the MMTV promoter', *Journal of Molecular Medicine*, vol. 74, pp.711-24.

Carrington, E.A. and Jones, R.S. (1996), 'The Drosophila Enhancer of zeste Gene Encodes a Chromosomal Protein: Examination of Wild-Type and Mutant Protein Distribution', *Development*, vol. 122, pp.4073-83.

Crick, F.H.C. (1958), 'On Protein Synthesis', *Symposium of the Society for Experimental Biology*, pp.138-63.

Hubbard, R and Wald, E. (1997), *Exploding the Gene Myth: How Genetic Information is Produced and Manipulated by Scientists, Physicians, Employers, Insurance Companies, Educators and Law Enforcers*, Boston, Beacon Press.

Kay, L.E. (1993), *The Molecular Vision of Life: Caltech, the Rockefeller Foundation and the Rise of the New Biology*, New York, Oxford University Press.

Keller, E. (1995), *Refiguring Life: Metaphors of Twentieth Century Biology*, New York, Columbia University Press.

Lander, E.S. and Weinberg, R.A. (2000), 'Genomics: Journey to the Center of Biology', *Science*, vol. 287, pp.1777-82.

Levins, R. and Lewontin, R. (1985), *The Dialectical Biologist*, Cambridge, MA, Harvard University Press.

Lewontin, R.C. (1992), *Biology as Ideology: the Doctrine of DNA*, Toronto, House of Anansi Press.

Lippman, A. (1991), 'Prenatal Genetic Testing and Screening: Constructing Needs and Reinforcing Inequities', *American Journal of Law and Medicine*, vol. 17, pp.15-50.

Loo, S. and Rine, J (1995), 'Silencing and Heritable Domains of Gene Expression', *Annual Review of Cell Developmental Biology*, vol. 11, pp.19-48.

Nelkin, D. (1995), *Selling Science: How the Press Covers Science and Technology*. Revised Edition, New York, W.H. Freeman and Co.

Nelkin, D. and Lindee, M.S. (1995), *The DNA Mystique: The Gene as Cultural Icon*, New York, W.H. Freeman and Co.

Olby, R.C. (1994), *The Path to the Double Helix: the Discovery of DNA*, New York, Dover Publications.

Sarkar, S. (1998), 'Forty Years Under the Central Dogma', *Trends in Biochemical Sciences*, pp.311-16.

Saul, J.R. (1995), *The Unconscious Civilization*, Toronto, House of Anansi Press.

Strohman, R.C. (1997), 'The Coming Kuhnian Revolution in Biology', *Nature Biotechnology*, vol. 5, pp.194-200.

Watson, J.D. (1965), *The Molecular Biology of the Gene*. W.A. Benjamin.

Watson, J.D. (1968), *The Double Helix: A Personal Account of the Discovery of the Structure of DNA*, New York, Mentor Books.

Watson, J.D. (1993), 'Looking Forward', *Gene*, vol. 135, pp.309-15.

Watson, J.D. and Crick, F.H.C. (1953), 'Molecular Structure of Nucleic Acids', *Nature*, vol. 171, p.737.

Wilson, E.O. *Sociobiology: The New Synthesis*, Cambridge, MA, Harvard University Press.

Chapter 10

Gene Manipulation, Psychology and Molecular Biology

Maurice K.D. Schouten

Leaping from molecules to mind

Molecular memory

In previous chapters, the use of gene therapy for medical reasons, and its possible implications have been examined. In this chapter, I focus on the role of genes in psychological and behavioral traits, in particular intelligence, learning and memory. Here the deterministic case may seem particularly strong, but not everyone finds this objectionable. Indeed, if major scientific journals like *Science* or *Nature* are to be believed, such a marriage of psychology and molecular biology is a match made in heaven.

Hardly a week passes without the announcement, to a suitable fanfare, of a new link between some behavioral trait and a specific gene or combination of genes. In December 1999, *Science* published its annual Top Ten list of most important scientific advances of the previous twelve months. Molecular biology occurs no less than four times, thereby once more emphasising that this may indeed be the Biology Century. The list is topped by research into stem cells, but one of the runners-up is research into the formation of what might be called *molecular memory*. For instance, Joe Tsien and his associates reported, in a September 1999 issue of *Nature*, of a genetically engineered 'brainier mouse' which outperformed its 'normal' (not modified) cousins on a battery of problem-solving tasks. In their words, this suggests that what they have discovered is the 'unifying mechanism underlying a variety of associative learning and memory' (Tang, Shimizu, Dube, Rampon, Kerchner, Zhuo, Liu, and Tsien, 1999, p.68). The idea behind such experiments in molecular biology is that research at the level of molecules may explain a mixed set of phenomena that one finds at the level of behavior. Yet despite the buzz, the truth may well be that many of these interlevel connections between genes and behavioral traits should be interpreted with caution. The assumptions and implications of the 'molecular memory' line of research in behavioral genetics will be the primary focus in this paper. More specifically, it will be asked whether this particular research program is capable of sustaining a *reductionistic* interpretation.

Molecular behavioral genetics

New molecular techniques have become available that allow behavioral geneticists to go beyond the statistical notion of the *heritability* of traits. Such techniques make it possible to make inferences with respect to the nature of the causal path from genotype to phenotype (Wahlsten, 1999; Wolf, 1995). Hence, these methods give the impression of being capable of building bridges between the neurosciences and the sciences of behavior. Tsien's experiments with the 'Doogie'[1] strain of mouse provide a case in point. They made the headlines of every self-respecting newspaper and magazine, inspiring talk of 'intelligence genes', 'genius genes', 'memory genes', and 'smart genes' and feeding speculations about memory-boosting and intelligence-enhancing pills and about gene therapies to fight various brain disorders such as Alzheimer's disease and schizophrenia. Even though the original publications do not usually give in to such wild speculation, talk of 'genes for' may still easily fuel interpretations of genetic research in terms of reductionism. As a first pass, *genetic reductionism* is the claim that when more and more is learnt about our genetic make-up (and the supposedly homologous genetic material in animals such as mice), more and more is understood about the relevant phenotypic (e.g., behavioral) traits, *because these phenotypic traits are determined (precoded, programmed, and so on) by the genotype*. That is, it argues from the *ontogenic primacy* of the genome to the conclusion that in the final analysis it is the genes that really count, ontologically and explanatorily speaking; it is the genes that *really* make a difference. Thus, reductionism may be seen to revive in the new and vibrant molecules-based behavioral genetics.

In particular, the analysis of learning and memory at the molecular level offers, as Kandel and his colleagues say, 'surprising reductionist possibilities' (Kandel, Schwartz, and Jessell, 1995, p.685). Certain genetic techniques (on which more below) allow neuroscientists and behavioral geneticists to break into the causal chains between genotype and phenotype, thus opening up new ways to approach the basic mechanisms underlying these cognitive functions with ever greater precision and specificity:

> A major advancement in our understanding of genes, their expression, and the structure of the proteins they encode has led to a better appreciation of the conservation of cellular function at the molecular level that now provides a common conceptual framework for several, previously unrelated, disciplines: cell biology, biochemistry, development, immunology, and cellular neurobiology. A parallel and potentially equally profound unification is occurring between cognitive psychology, the science of the mind, and neural science. (Bailey, Bartsch and Kandel, 1996, p.13445)

The genetic techniques used to dissect learning and memory are thought to 'bridge molecular mechanisms to cognition' (Kandel, et al., 1995, p.685, p.686). The rhetoric has it that we may finally be able to 'begin to bridge the gap in understanding how the genes control neuronal function and how neuronal function, in turn, controls behavior' (Mayford, Abel and Kandel, 1995, p.146). This may imply that when all the molecular facts are in there may no longer be any point in talking about learning and memory qua *psychological* phenomena as learning and memory will be exhaustively *molecularized*. In that case, a specification of the relevant genetic material proves to be sufficiently powerful to account for each and every aspect of what are now considered to be psychological phenomena. On reductionistic interpretations, behavioral, neural, and mental traits originate in the genetic material. After the 'gene-ification' of neural science (Routtenberg, 1996), there will be bottom-up reductionism: the genotype *determines*, and thereby exhausts, the phenotype, learning and memory not excluded. Hence, these traits are *reducible* to their genetic origins. In order to evaluate these claims, let us move on to a brief discussion of the 'molecular memory' hypothesis, without plunging too deep into the complex lingo of genetics and neuroscience.

Gene modification and the dissection of learning and memory

According to Eric Kandel and his co-workers, long-term memory requires the synthesis of new mRNA or new proteins and the growth of new synaptic contacts (Kandel, et al., 1995, p.671ff.). The complex biochemical cascade that is responsible for this looks roughly as follows. One class of membrane protein, namely the NMDA receptor channel, in particular in certain areas of the hippocampus, is thought to function as a kind of molecular gatekeeper: it controls the influx of Ca^{2+} in the postsynaptic neuron. The NMDA receptor opens only when two coincident conditions are met: (1) the neurotransmitter glutamate, released by a neighbouring neuron, must bind to the receptor and (2) the Mg^{2+} block that normally keeps the receptor closed must be relieved through a depolarization of the neuron. Once the calcium flows in *long-term potentiation* (or LTP), i.e. the enhancement of synaptic transmission, is initiated (see e.g., Malenka and Nicoll, 1999). Increased cytosolic calcium levels lead to both a short-term and a long-term process. The latter process is initiated by the activation of adenylyl cyclase which is responsible for an increase in the second messenger cyclic AMP (cAMP) in the neuron. Now cAMP activates the cAMP-dependent protein kinase A (PKA) by attaching to its regulatory subunit which results in a release of its catalytic subunit. PKA translocates to the nucleus of the hippocampal neuron. Here it induces phosphorylation of certain transcriptional regulatory proteins that bind to cyclic AMP regulatory elements (CREB). CREB increases the expression of a number of different effector genes that code for a number of different proteins. One such class of produced proteins is responsible for the activation of protein kinase A so that phosphorylation is constantly maintained in the nucleus of the nerve cell.

Until recently, these molecular mechanisms underlying learning and memory were largely studied by means of pharmacological studies based on the ability of some pharmacological agents (e.g., NMDA receptor antagonists) to block LTP and to compromise learning (as determined in some behavioral test, e.g., the Morris water maze). These experiments are fairly limited though, because they are fraught with a number of severe difficulties (Mayford, et al., 1995, p.142; see also Schouten and Looren de Jong, 1999). Since the late 1980s, other techniques have become available that look promising as a means to study the molecular basis of cognitive functions. These techniques, derived from molecular biology, are based on the manipulation of neuronal structures (such as the NMDA receptor channel or its subunits) by modification of the genome (in model organisms like mice). This methodology is now employed by Kandel's group and other groups of investigators (e.g., Tonegawa's, Tsien's) to shed a light on the processes that are involved in learning and memory (Mayford, et al., 1995).

Two basic strategies to create genetically engineered animals (in particular mice) can be distinguished, *viz.* (1) *transgenesis* and (2) *gene-targeting* (e.g., Wehner, Bowers, and Paylor, 1996). The transgenic approaches refers to the introduction of exogenous or foreign DNA into the mouse genome. The *gene targeting* approach was pioneered by, among others, Mario Capecchi (1989a, 1989b, 1994). Gene targeting involves the replacement (or inactivation) of a gene on a chromosome by homologous recombination in embryonic stem (ES) cells. The ablation of the gene results in phenotypic alteration of, for instance, processes that involve learning and memory. As a consequence of the genetic treatment, the gene product is missing, and this, in combination with these mice performing badly on certain behavioral tests, allows one to draw conclusions with regard to both the functional roles of the disrupted gene and of the physiological processes that are supposed to be normally dependent on its expression.[2] In some experiments, the *CREB* gene in a specific strain of mice was inactivated ('knocked out'). When these *CREB* knockout mice were tested, they proved to be considerably hampered in their ability to store information (often *spatial* information) over longer periods of time compared to the wild-type controls. This has suggested the hypothesis that CREB function is critical for the formation of long-term memories. In fact, it has been suggested that *CREB* may be a 'learning gene' (Greenspan, 1995, p.78).

But other genes are likely to be involved. In particular, genes that are more directly involved in the development of NMDA receptors. The aforementioned work by Tsien's Princeton lab is a case in point. Their experiments with genetically manipulated mice, this time with genes *added* (namely, genes coding for a specific subunit of the NMDA receptor, named NR2B) rather than deleted, led to the development of smarter mice rather than dumber ones (Tang, et al., 2000; cf. Bliss, 1999). Overexpression of the NR2B subunit led to a great enhancement of LTP and to a superior performance on a number of behavioral (including non-spatial) tasks requiring learning and memory.

These findings, then, are supposed to vindicate the 'molecular memory' hypothesis: the molecular processes underlying NMDA-mediated LTP are crucial for learning and memory. Because of its capacity to act as a 'coincidence detector', the NMDA receptor, and the process of LTP it mediates, is thought to be crucially involved in learning and memory. Gene manipulation may ultimately provide the master key to the Hebb learning rule which, to put it colloquially, states that '*When cells fire together, they wire together*'.

Both methodologies, gene deletion and gene addition, hold the assumption in common that genes are directly causally related to traits at the phenotypic levels, so that tampering with these genes affects the traits they are linked with. Whether this counts as genetic reductionism, however, remains to be seen.

Geneticism and developmentalism

Geneticism

According to genetic reductionists, for *real* explanations, one should go molecular. For reductionism to work, there is no need to resort to classical reductionism (with its talk about laws, statements, identities, theories, and so on). In general, it will suffice to unveil singular causal chains by bringing out how observable phenotypic traits and their functions are related to (i.e., determined or controlled by) molecular processes (Rosenberg, 1997, p.462). Tracing out such causal paths from genotype to phenotype may result in so-called 'single-plot stories'. According to *genetic reductionism* in its most simplistic form, genetic properties are causally sufficient for phenotypic traits. Although a causal sufficiency requirement will, by most biologists, be rejected as too strong, the popularity of metaphors like 'genetic program', 'genetic blueprint', and 'mastermolecule' (Oyama, 1985; Van der Weele, 1999) indicates that many biologists do typically assign some kind of causal priority to the genome. Such a view implies a kind of *computational reductionism*: the development of an embryo can in principle be computed from, and explained by, a full specification of the genome present in a cell (Rosenberg, 1997). The idea of genetic control that is behind computational reductionism of course goes back to Francis Crick's formulation of the *Central Dogma* of molecular biology: there is a one-way flow of information from DNA via RNA to proteins.[3] It may be thought that, for instance, psychological processes are in the end completely controlled by what goes on at the level of molecules. This interpretation may derive some plausibility from the methodologies involving gene manipulation. However, the problems with, in particular, the gene targeting approach are many (Gerlai, 1996a, 1996b; Routtenberg, 1996), and these problems suggest that an alternative interpretation may be what is required.

Developmentalism

Some authors, writing on the methodology of gene targeting, have stated that the mutant mouse is not just a mouse with only one local protein missing, namely the one coded for by the missing allele, but that they are entirely different from how they would have been without the mutation. They are 'reactionisms' (Routtenberg, 1995), that is, in the course of its development it has *actively*, not passively, responded to the mutation. There may, for instance, be *compensatory processes* at work due to the expression of other, related genes for the specific gene that was deleted, thereby *masking* the effects of the null mutation (Crawley, 1996). *Pleiotropy* is a factor that makes interpretation difficult. Multiple phenotypic effects may be observed, because of the gene's absence throughout the CNS of the developing animal (Crawley, 1996; Mayford, et al., 1995, p.142; Wilson and Tonegawa, 1997, p.102). Further, there is also a problem concerning genetic context, because the effects of other genes (strain background) are overlooked: 'genes act in concert and the disruption of genetic material, let it be as targeted as one would like it to be, will always lead to a complex systemic response' (Gerlai, 1996a, p.189). Polymorphism in the genetic background may cause large neurobiological or behavioral differences (Gerlai, 1996b). Gerlai documents that, for instance, in mouse strain 129 passivity and defects in the corpus callosum have been observed. Different strains of mice perform differently (Lathe, 1996). These problems indicate that the danger is real that too much is claimed on the basis of too little (see also Culp, 1997). These problems suggests that an interpretation of the new behavioral genetics in terms of genetic (or computational) reductionism is implausible. A different interpretation is given by *developmentalism*.

According to developmentalism, computational reductionism is inadequate to account for the complexity of organismic development. Developmentalists hold that there are not only causal pathways from DNA to phenotype, but also pathways from supragenetic resources (e.g., the cytoplasm) back to the genetic material. Individual development can only be understood if the many interactions between the nodes of an enormous causal network, stretching out from genes via cellular structures and organs to the extra-organismic environment, is taken into account. Central to developmentalism is the concept of *parity* (Schaffner, 1998). It argues against the primacy of the genome. Genes, according to developmentalism, are not in any sense *causally, informationally, and explanatorily* priviliged as Crick's Central Dogma suggested. On the reductionist's picture, the information requisite for development is present in the molecular structure of the genes. The causal processes of development are initiated at this genetic level. From here the organism develops linearly. Hence, ontogenetic processes must ultimately be accounted for in terms of DNA. These assumptions are questioned by developmentalism. The role of emergence and self-organization in ontogeny is emphasised. Individual development is an historical process in which each new state (and function) of the developmental system builds upon previously existing states (and functions) of an interactive network (Gottlieb, 1992, pp.159-160). There is an inexorable intertwining of causes and their effects. According to developmentalists, there is not only causal, but also *informational* parity: genes have little meaning by themselves; they rely on a context of cellular, extracellular, and exogenous interactants. Information is not encrypted in the DNA. Rather, information is constructed on the basis of numerous, not just genetic, resources. The developmentalist concludes that 'because of the molecular and biochemical interactions producing the phenotype, it appears to be arbitrary to give the genetic part a priviliged rank' (Wolf, 1995, p.132). Causal and informational parity suggest that there is *explanatory* parity as well, according to developmentalism. It is hard to see how, on this picture, gene targeting can have any special relevance for the study of learning and memory. Such cognitive processes must be the outcome of extremely complex and interactional processes taking place in an enormous causal web. In the following, I will suggest that although developmentalists are right to claim that an interpretation in terms of computational reductionism is unwarranted, there is still a sense in which the new behavioral genetics gives valuable information.

Localization and decomposition

Neurophysiological decomposition and genetic localization

Because of its attempts to infer brain function from local deletions, gene targeting is similar in certain respects to the study of brain lesions. In fact, it has been dubbed a case of *microphrenology* (Crusio, 1996). Developmentalism rightly insists that there are all kinds of qualifications to be made in interpreting genotype/phenotype relationships. Development is the product of complex causal interplay, even penetrating deeply into the environment. Still, the success of experimental paradigms like the gene targeting approach suggests that the developmentalists' holism may be too radical. Although the reduction of traits to genes, given the enormous complexity of developmental processes, is implausible, the new behavioral genetics does, in a way, appear to advance our understanding of higher-level processes like learning and memory. In the remainder of this essay, I will explore a different interpretation of research at the interface of (molecular) genetics and psychology.

According to Bechtel and Richardson (1993), complex systems can be understood as enormously expanded, high-dimensional problem spaces. Because we cannot take each and every variable into account, we need to have some well-tried search strategies that constrain alternative interpretations of the way a system performs its task or function. Bechtel and Richardson explore two basic research tools to get explanatory grip on complex systems, namely *decomposition* and *localization*, which are, as history shows, effective ways to guide our scientific searches through these problem spaces. In a decomposition, system functions are analysed into component functions. Localization means attempting to pin down the structural parts that are mechanically responsible for higher-level functions, for instance, those found in a decomposition. Gene targeting may invite an interpretation in terms of localization and decomposition. The functions of learning and memory, for instance, may be decomposed (*top-down*) into various subfunctions, such as short-term and long-term memory, habituation, sensitization, and classical conditioning. Further, from the viewpoint of molecular genetics, *bottom-up* decomposition is at least as important as the following quote suggests: '[t]he power of genetics is its ability to dissect the sequence of steps involved in a particular physiological pathway' (Mayford, et al., 1995, p.146). Just as phrenology in the 19th century and later lesion studies led to the identification of brain areas directly involved in mental functions, these subfunctions of learning and memory, and the neurophysiological mechanisms that implement them, may now via the method of gene lesioning, be localized in the activity of specific genes. Thus, gene targeting may be interpreted as a way to link a phenotypic trait such a memory to a specific gene. That is, the higher-level trait is localized in that gene. If successful, the gene targeting approach identifies the *locus of control* for development.

That such a direct link between genes and phenotypic traits is possible is contested, as we saw, by developmentalists. They would argue that direct genetic localization of behavioral or cognitive traits presents an oversimplification. In the case of development, one encounters what Bechtel and Richardson call an 'emergent' or 'integrated' mechanism. As the number of components in a system and the interactions between them, increases, the heuristics of decomposition and localization may eventually fail. In the case of really complex systems, there is *distributed control*: the outcomes of development depend on interactions between relatively homogeneous components. In the case of a truly integrated system, localization and decomposition may fall widely of the mark, because the processes in these networks are, as Bechtel and Richardson express it, 'multiply constrained' (1993, p.125). If there is any substance to the claim that the causal processes underlying learning and memory constitute such a multiply constrained, integrated network, with control distributed over many or even all of its nodes, the gene manipulation methodology may lose much of its attraction.

The 'how' and 'why' of development

The notion of a locus of control is potentially ambiguous in the case of behavioral genetics. I will argue that one needs to distinguish between the locus of causal control and the locus of informational control. By localizing the origin of a phenotypic trait in a specific gene, one pins down the *informational*, but not (as the developmentalists show) the *causal* locus of control. This means that the gene targeting approach can be seen as providing us with valuable information, without closing one's eyes for the enormous causal complexity of the processes involved.

Kenneth Schaffner has provided a thorough analysis of the developmentalists' claims in the context of investigations of the genome of the nematode *C. elegans*. This resulted in a number of important conclusions. In Schaffner's view, developmentalists are certainly right to emphasise that organismic development involves a tangle of causal factors, and that therefore a simple-minded form of genetic reductionism must be wrong. Pleiotropy, plasticity, and environmental context effects are ubiquitous. This suggests that there is *causal* parity. However, *explanatory and informational* parity do not follow, according to Schaffner. Although genetic factors are causally on a par with extragenetic factors, the genome must be considered informationally priviliged. The 'Central Dogma' is correct in essence, according to Schaffner (1998, p.234). And because the genome is informationally priviliged, explanations in terms of genetic resources must be considered explanatorily priviliged (at least in some contexts of inquiry).

Often what is demanded is not a specification of all causal factors that contributed to a trait. It is not *how* questions, but *why* questions that are often the most interesting and revealing questions, and 'why' questions are always posed against a fixed background of causal factors. In answering a 'why' question, a gene (or complex of genes) may still be given explanatory priority, because it is *selected* to produce some phenotypic trait. 'Genes for' may be identified, although they are only 'genes for' relative to a given causal background (Clark, 1998a, 1998b). Given a fixed ecological backdrop, the genetic material functions as a primary *locus of plasticity*, because a change in the gene(s) would result in a change in the phenotypic trait. Holding constant the causal (i.e., the ecological and developmental) background, parts of the genome can be singled out as the factor that (primarily) causes or *represents* the trait on the basis of the fact (or conjecture) that it was the specific gene complex that was selected to replicate the phenotypic traits. Genes are *designed* or *selected* mechanisms to ensure parent-offspring stability: in virtue of their representational capacities, the genetic material has the function of bringing about a particular phenotypic consequence. Other causal (e.g., environmental) factors involved in the production of phenotypic traits are *not* so designed.

> Consider a facultatively desert-adapted shrub; a shrub whose leaf structure and shape reduces water loss if grown in arid environments. Both aridity and the shrub's genome are necessary for that shrub's adaptive response to the environment. But that genome only exists because of the causal path (in that environment) from genome to desert-resistant shrub. By contrast, the aridity of the environment exists independently of the causal path (in that genetic environment) from arid conditions to desert adapted shrub. One element of the developmental matrix exists only because of its role in the production of the plant lineage phenotype. That is why it has the function of producing that phenotype, and hence why it represents that phenotype. (Sterelny, Smith, and Dickison, 1996, pp.388-389)

Both aridity and genome correlate or co-vary with desert-adapted shrub, but it is only the genome that, in virtue of its selectional history, can be said to have the function of replicating shrub structure and shape; the aridity-shrub connection is merely (asymmetrically) dependent upon the genome-shrub connection.

Against a stable backdrop of ecological, notably climatic (namely, arid) and developmental conditions, the desert shrub's genome is the principal difference-maker, the principal locus of plasticity. Altering the plant's genetic material would alter its adaptive phenotypic properties (namely, its desert-resistance). The gene set exists because of its role in the bringing about of the plant's capacities to hold water. So, whereas the genome is dependent for its existence on the causal pathway between genome and phenotypic outcome, there is no such dependence (in this particular genetic environment) of aridity on the causal nexus between aridity and the trait. On this account, one is still allowed to speak of 'genes coding for traits' although this notion must be relativized to a set of normal ecological background conditions (Sterelny and Kitcher, 1988). Though genes may not be *causally* priviliged, they may be *explanatorily* prioritized in some contexts of investigation, because they function as information-carriers (see also Wheeler and Clark, 1999). A different way to put the same point is that one may say that although there is no *causal* locus of control (i.e., the causal work is distributed over numerous nodes in the causal network), there is an *informational* locus of control. Because the genome functions as an informational locus of control, it may be said that at least for certain types of inquiry, the genome is explanatorily more relevant than the other, non-genetic factors causally involved. Talking about 'genes for' constitutes a (context-relative) way to interpret what goes on in these labyrinthine, multiply constrained webs.

The new molecular behavioral genetics can be interpreted in this light. Through techniques such as gene targeting and QTL analysis, causal relations can be established between the molecular and phenotypic levels, more specifically, the levels of mind, brain, and behavior. The warning must however be heeded that these types of research can easily result in overly ambitious, too reductionistic or deterministic interpretations. However, the claim that gene-targeting techniques used to dissect learning and memory can 'bridge molecular mechanisms to cognition' (Kandel, et al., 1995, p.686) must not be read reductionistically. That said, however, this does not mean that behavioral genetics becomes worthless. On the contrary, it may still be possible to trace, through these tangled paths of causality, important factors that contribute to the emergence of behavioral traits.

Conclusion

An exclusive focus on the level of molecules is not likely to take us very far in explaining what learning and memory is. There is more to these phenomena than what one finds at the lowest levels of investigation. Deterministic single-plot stories are not likely to suffice. In that sense, there are no learning or memory genes. Research in behavioral genetics does not offer complete molecular explanations, but rather local bridges between different domains of investigation. Investigation of the molecular bricks and mortar of memory by tinkering with genes may be fruitful, but it must not be forgotten that the psychological level will also be required. Behavioral genetics invites an interpretation in terms of *explanatory pluralism* (see also Schouten and Looren de Jong, in press). Multilevel analysis is needed 'to coordinate inquiry and to seek mutual intelligibility' (Oyama, 1985, p.154). There are many causal processes at work in development and many of them are in the domain of psychology. Whereas information may only flow upward (contra developmentalism), causal control flows in both directions (contra reductionism). Further, psychology will be needed to clarify the *functions* of learning and memory (Schouten and Looren de Jong, 1999). Hence, bottom-up and top-down approaches will both be necessary.

Notes

1   The strain is called Doogie after the precocious lead character of the television series *Doogie Howser, M.D.*

2   Normally, the knockout procedure starts with the cloning of the gene of interest. This gene is altered in line with the intentions and interests of the researcher. Subsequently, the altered DNA sequence (*targeting vector*) is brought into the cell nucleus of isolated

pluripotent ES cells. This is done by way of, for instance, microinjection or electroporation (Wehner et al., 1996). The targeting vector searches through the nucleotide sequences of the genome until it finds its *target*. The actual targeting of the vector DNA to specific chromosomal sites is effected through homologous recombination. Ideally, then, the targeting vector lines up next to its target, and takes its place. Thus, a null allele is created. The cells are incorporated by microinjection into a mouse embryo at the (preimplantation) blastocyst stage. When all goes well, the whole procedure results in transgenic (or knockout) mice. This brief overview of the knockout procedure was based largely on three articles by Capecchi (1989a, 1989b, 1994).

3   Gene expression is a two-step process. First, messenger RNA (mRNA) is *transcribed* upon DNA templates. Second, this mRNA travels from the nucleus of the cell to the cytoplasm where it is *translated* into the amino acid sequences that constitute a protein.

References

Bailey, C.H., Bartsch, D. and Kandel, E.R. (1996), 'Towards a molecular definition of long-term memory storage', *Proceedings of the National Academy of Sciences USA*, vol. 93, pp.13445-13452.

Bliss, T.V.P. (1999), 'Young receptors make smart mice', *Nature*, vol. 401, pp.25-27.

Capecchi, M.R. (1989a), 'Altering the genome by homologous recombination', *Science*, vol. 244, pp.1288-1292.

Capecchi, M.R. (1989b), 'The new mouse genetics: Altering the genome by gene targeting', *Trends in Genetics*, vol. 5, pp.70-76.

Capecchi, M.R.(1994), 'Targeted gene replacement', *Scientific American*, vol. 270, March, pp.34-41.

Clark, A. (1998a), 'Time and mind', *Journal of Philosophy*, vol. 95, pp.354-376.

Clark, A. (1998b), 'Twisted tales: Causal complexity and cognitive scientific explanation', *Minds and Machines*, vol. 8, pp.79-99.

Crawley, J.N. (1996), 'Unusual behavioral phenotypes of inbred mouse strains', *Trends in Neurosciences*, vol. 19, pp.181-182.

Crusio, W.E. (1996), 'Gene-targeting studies: New methods, old problems', *Trends in Neurosciences*, vol. 19, pp.186-187.

Culp, S. (1997), 'Establishing genotype/phenotype relationships: Gene targeting as an experimental approach', *Philosophy of Science*, vol. 64, S268-S278.

Gerlai, R. (1996a), 'Gene targeting in neuroscience: The systemic approach', *Trends in Neuroscience*, vol. 19, pp.188-189.

Gerlai, R. (1996b), 'Gene-targeting studies of mammalian behavior: Is it the mutation or the background phenotype?', *Trends in Neurosciences*, vol. 19, pp.177-181.

Greenspan, R.J. (1995), 'Understanding the genetic construction of behavior', *Scientific American*, vol. 272, April, pp.74-79.

Kandel, E.R., Schwartz, J.H. and Jessell, T.M. (1995), *Essentials of neural science and behavior*, Norwalk, CT, Appleton and Lange.

Lathe, R. (1996), 'Mice, gene targeting and behaviour: More than just genetic background', *Trends in Neurosciences*, vol. 19, pp.183-186.

Malenka, R.C. and Nicoll, R.A. (1999), 'Long-term potentiation: A decade of progress?' *Science*, vol. 285, pp.1870-1874.

Mayford, M., Abel, T. and Kandel, E.R. (1995), 'Transgenic approaches to cognition', *Current Opinion in Neurobiology*, vol. 5, pp.141-148.

Oyama, S. (1985), *The ontogeny of information*, Cambridge, Cambridge University Press.

Rosenberg, A. (1997), 'Reductionism redux: Computing the embryo', *Biology and Philosophy*, vol. 12, pp.445-470.

Routtenberg, A. (1996), 'Reverse piedpiperase: Is the knockout mouse leading neuroscientists to a watery end?', *Trends in Neurosciences*, vol. 19, pp.471-472.

Schaffner, K.F. (1998), 'Genes, behavior, and developmental emergentism: One process, indivisible?', *Philosophy of Science*, vol. 65, pp.209-252.

Schouten, M.K.D. and Looren de Jong, H. (1999), 'Reduction, elimination, and levels: The case of the LTP-learning link', *Philosophical Psychology*, vol. 12, pp.237-262.

Schouten, M.K.D. and Looren de Jong, H. (in press), 'Pluralism and heuristic identification: Some explorations in behavioral genetics', *Theory and Psychology*.

Sterelny, K. and Kitcher, P. (1988), 'The return of the gene', *Journal of Philosophy*, vol. 85, pp.339-361.

Sterelny, K., Kitcher, P., Smith, K.C., and Dickison, M. (1996) 'The extended replicator', *Biology and Philosophy*, vol. 11, pp.377-404.

Tang, Y.-P., Shimizu, E., Dube, G.R., Rampon, C., Kerchner, G., Zhuo, M., Liu, G. and Tsien, J.Z. (1999), 'Genetic enhancement of learning and memory in mice', *Nature*, vol. 401, pp.63-69.

Tsien, J.Z. (2000), 'Building a brainier mouse', *Scientific American*, vol. 282, pp.42-48.

Van der Weele, C. (1999), *Images of development: Environmental causes in ontogeny*, Albany, NY, SUNY Press.

Wahlsten, D. (1999), 'Single-gene influences on brain and behavior', *Annual Review of Psychology*, vol. 50, pp.599-624.

Wehner, J.M., Bowers, B., J. and Paylor, R. (1996), 'The use of null mutant mice to study complex learning and memory processes', *Behavior Genetics*, vol. 26, pp.301-312.

Wheeler, M. and Clark, A. (1999), 'Genic representation: Reconciling content and causal complexity', *British Journal for the Philosophy of Science*, vol. 50, pp.103-135.

Wilson, M.A. and Tonegawa, S. (1997), 'Synaptic plasticity, place cells and spatial memory: Study with second generation knockouts', *Trends in Neurosciences*, vol. 20, pp.102-106.

Wolf, U. (1995), 'The genetic contribution to the phenotype', *Human Genetics*, vol. 95, pp.127-148.

Chapter 11

Patenting Human DNA

Andy Miah

The scientific advances described in earlier chapters have inevitably triggered a response in the world of business and economics, and in this chapter I consider the recent activities of the American company, Celera Genomics, which aims to obtain patent rights for aspects of the human genome. This brings into question whether life, indeed human life, should belong to anyone or anybody. It raises, too, the further question as to how this new information will be used.

The issue of DNA ownership has not been neglected within bioethics and biolegal studies. Articles and books in these areas invoke concepts of human dignity, objectifying life, and life as a consumer product in the context of patenting DNA. The main part of such ethical investigations has been related to agriculture or non-human organisms. This is not surprising given the immediacy of technologies such as the patenting of the cloning procedure that was used to create Dolly the sheep. Central to these concerns are the implications such patenting has for the development of scientific research and the, supposedly, vulgar franchising (and likely exploitation) of human body parts. However, it remains unclear whether the patenting of DNA does actually count as owning life and whether this somewhat emotive response to patenting is justified. Thus, it is important to clarify the significance of patenting DNA and to outline what it would actually involve.

Numerous forms of patenting biological processes can be considered as morally problematic. The development of new drugs or therapeutic medical techniques, which might be dependent on the sequencing of a DNA strand, might also be of interest to scientists wishing to obtain patents. However, of particular interest in this chapter is the patenting of human DNA that might, some day, be used to (pro)create new human life or contribute to the sustainability of any human life. What, in particular, might be the implications for an individual if his or her genetic heritage is owned by an organisation, rather than having been passed down by biological parents? Such circumstances appear unsettling since it seems to amount to manufacturing a life that a business company might have created. I would argue, however, that such reductionism is not sufficient to discard the moral acceptability of patenting human DNA. Rather, it distracts us from the more significant social implications of this prospect. This is not to dismiss the philosophical implications as unimportant. Rather, it is to acknowledge the proper content of philosophical implications about patenting human DNA.

This lack of clarity begs the question of what is the moral significance of owning such material and to what degree one's identity is comprised by one's genetic heritage – if, indeed, it is. For, it is not immediately clear how the patenting of human DNA could pose any threat at all to any individual. Undoubtedly, there is much controversy about this matter and intuitive appeals to human dignity, identity, and the sanctity of human life are often given as reasons for not patenting human DNA. Yet, much of this dialogue seems rather a sentimental appeal to claims about our humanness, as if this is some fixed concept that humans must possess. Thus, it is vital to clarify the credibility of such arguments and to comprehend the actual threat that patenting raises. The mere fact that a blueprint of the human genome could reveal something about a particular individual does not seem, necessarily, problematic. Yet, the way such information is used and made available to interested parties does have implications that are morally questionable. Should, for example, the owners of particular aspects of the human genome be entitled to sell this information to research companies seeking such morally worthy objectives as vaccines for diseases? Equally, should such patenting be made available to companies who seek to commercialise life, privatise organ donorship, and treat medical care as an industry to be exploited wherever possible? If not, then what claim does the former have above the latter that makes its moral evaluation acceptable?

Integral to the distaste about patenting life is the prospect of trading human life – the combining of money with human dignity. Indeed, if one is forced to state the strongest, most intuitive argument against such technology, it would be this. Arguably, where the concept of owning biological life, particularly human life, is invoked, one is immediately drawn to Huxleyan images of a very inhuman, unpleasant society where lives are automated, uncreative, and disturbingly lacking in this elusive quality of humanness. In his *Brave New World,* Huxley's descriptions are unequivocal, and the human individuals are savage and ungainly. In contrast is a perception of life that is creative, emotional, passionate, and spiritual and it remains the reaction of many people to genetic technologies.

Evidence of such disaffection has appeared most recently from the emergence of *Ron's Angels*, a company set up for the auctioning of female eggs and male sperm to infertile couples seeking 'exceptional' children. Whilst numerous companies of this kind now exist, *Ron's Angels* is interesting not simply for having arranged a standard and reasonable price for such genes; far from it. Rather, as indicated above, eggs and sperm are awarded to the highest bidder. One might argue that the method of auctioning is the most exploitative of methods of purchase. This might be contested by saying that, with auctioning, nobody pays more than that which they believe to be a fair price. However, such a claim fails to recognise the circumstances of the bidding parties, who, in this case, are likely to be particularly vulnerable, since it would seem that such donations would be necessary only where individuals or couples could not have children of their own for whatever reasons. Thus, such persons are in a situation of dependency upon the new reproductive technologies and products. One might respond to and legitimate these circumstances by arguing that such people need not use such a company, since they could seek these donations through more conventional medical services. However, it is my contention that the appeal of superficially super-human or 'perfect' genes is particularly attractive where the ease of receiving them is very straightforward. It is this reality that lends strength to concluding that the practice is morally problematic.

Though limited in choice of stock (there are really very few donors), this pioneering genetic supermarket offers a very simply rationale for utilising its services. It claims that it is simply seeking to promote choice, providing prospective parents the opportunity to purchase the contemporary social assets of intelligence and beauty (and, to appear more legitimate, health). The introduction to the company states that,

> Beauty is its own reward. This is the first society to truly comprehend how important beautiful genes are to our evolution. Just watch television and you will see that we are only interested in looking at beautiful people ... our society is obsessed with youth and beauty. As our society grows older, we inevitably look to youth and beauty. The billion dollar cosmetic industry, including cosmetic surgery is proof of our obsession with beauty.

> What is the significance of beauty? It has been reported that young babies prefer to look at a symmetrical face, rather that an asymmetrical one. Beautiful people are usually given the job of selling to, and interacting with society. This continues throughout our adulthood. The act of creating better looking, or in some organisms, more disease resistant offspring (known as Genetic Modifications), has been taking place for hundreds of years. All genetic modifications serve to improve the shape, color and traits of the organism. 'Aroma and attractiveness is nature's shorthand for health and hardiness'. If you could increase the chance of reproducing beautiful children, and thus giving them an advantage in society, would you?

> Any gift such as beauty, intelligence, or social skills, will help your children in their quest for happiness and success (Harris, R., 1999).

From here, one begins to recognise the potential realisation of a manufactured future for the human species, with the next line of products being the genes (sperm or eggs) of athletes or professors. Indeed, recent news headlines reveal infertility couples seeking the eggs of Oxbridge students (Harlow and Gould, 1999). One can quite easily imagine how this can generate an immediate response of revulsion at the concept of owning life, given these practices.

Condemned by many infertility groups world wide, of all the applications of genetic technologies, this practice seems unequivocally repulsive for the simple reason that it has the effect of forcing the values of one generation upon another, thus stalling social change and the possibility of reflecting upon values. The prioritising of beauty or a particular version of intelligence in some of these enterprises and the inevitable projection of this value onto future generations, implicitly coerces the user into sharing these values. It forces one to consider that if, as a prospective parent, you do not recognise these assets and provide them for your children, then you will disadvantage your child. Thus, the message appeals to an enduring notion of wanting to provide the best future for one's child. Such inferences are alarming for, as in the case of the infertile couple, it seeks to manipulate the vulnerable. It also means, of course, that the procedures are available to others who are *not* infertile, but will use the available technology for eugenic goals.

Returning again to the patenting of human DNA, it is important to note, too, the legal implications of this process. From a legal position, whether the human genome should belong to anyone requires one to take a position on whether new life is seen as invention or discovery. It is necessary to establish whether the sequencing of DNA is, indeed, something that warrants a patent. The Patent Trading Office (PTO) deems that 'all genetically engineered multicellular living organisms, including animals, are potentially patentable' (cited in Rifken, 1998, p.44). Moreover, Donald J. Quigg, Commissioner of Patents and Trademarks in the USA, said that, 'patenting covered all but human beings as this would be against the Thirteenth Amendment to the Constitution, which forbids human slavery. This seems to entail, though, that genetically altered human embryos and fetuses as well as human genes, cell lines, tissues and organs are potentially patentable, and to leave open the possibility of patenting all of the separate parts, if not the whole, of a human being' (p.45). The requirements of being granted a patent on something are disturbingly straightforward and are as follows:

1   It must be novel (new).
2   It must not be obvious. Nothing can be patented in its natural state, including native varieties of plants or animals, or anything within the human body that has not been genetically modified. A customary use of a natural object cannot be patented either. A new or non-obvious 'use' of something occurring in nature is patentable, however.
3   It must have utility. 'Rube Goldberg' nonsense machines are not patentable. (British law, unlike U.S. law, does not require utility.) (Cited in Wertz, 1999.)

These details, it would seem then, do not preclude the patenting of human genetic material, despite the reluctance of patenting authorities to grant such rights in this age of uncertainty. So, let us now turn to some objections to the patenting of human DNA, drawing first from more general concerns about patenting biological material.

The issue of patenting raises numerous socio-economic concerns. These concerns in the case of plants and animals are discussed in detail in Part 3, but some preliminary remarks are relevant here. In the context of agriculture, for example, the fear that ownership will have a negative impact upon the sustainability of the third-world suggests a need for precaution in granting such patents (Reiss and Straughan, 1996). Nevertheless, there is an argument that genetic engineering and the patenting of modified strands of agricultural DNA, can allow a *greater* provision for third-world countries, where harsh climates and scarce resources limit people's survivability. Where new technology could be patented to enable the development of foods that could flourish in such environments, it seems desirable to promote this.

Nevertheless, the genetic engineering of foodstuffs does provoke concerns about the safety of the technology and the unknown long-term effects of human beings consuming these foods. Despite reassurance from scientists about the safety of these foods or, at least, the proximity of levels of safety to non-GM foods, many people continue to feel distrustful about science and medicine in this respect. In the case of biological organisms, the subject of patenting raises concerns over their treatment and some commentators argue that the patenting of animals and the creation of new life forms will generate a lack of respect for animals as sentient beings, of value in themselves (Holtug, 1998; Terragni, 1993). These critics fear that animals will be seen as products, owned and to be exploited. Here, however, I am concerned with the patenting of *human* DNA, though I believe we should take note of the application of patenting to other animal species when considering the ownership of aspects of the human genome and more generally, ownership of life and the autonomy of individuals.

Concerns about the patenting of human DNA are quite distinct, though there are some parallel issues that seem exaggerated due to aspects of the technology. Firstly, whilst the patenting system might be a necessary procedure to promote research in science and medicine, if such findings are patented, then such information – such discoveries or inventions – might not be used for the greatest good. This utilitarian perspective might not be justified, though it is undoubtedly of critical interest for the patenting system (Owen, 1995). Thus, for example, if a gene sequence was developed that could contribute to the prevention of various diseases, then, ideally, one would hope that this information would be made available to all those who might be able to develop it further. However, the patenting of such findings might limit their use only to those companies who are able to pay for the licensing rights. Consequently, it is reasonable to fear that patenting might have the negative effect of stifling research that would be for the greater good of human well-being.

While not denying the need to keep in mind practical objectives like this, I want here to contest the more general objection to patenting human DNA: that it will have the effect of devaluing human life and be an affront to human dignity. Such concerns have been discussed by a number of writers in relation to the Kantian principle of treating persons as ends in themselves rather than as means to the ends of other people.[1] However, in the context of patenting, I would suggest that these concerns are not warranted and that patenting human DNA does not present any such difficulties, since they are premised upon a misunderstanding of the patenting process and aspire to genocentric ideals that are not justified.

The claim about human dignity as threatened by patenting is based on a misunderstanding about types and levels, since the technology under question does not belong to a specific individual. Rather, the patenting of human DNA belongs to the human species and not to any individual member of that species. Thus, any claim about dignity premised upon the Kantian notion must be extended to encompass the dignity of a species rather than any member of it. Such a concept is problematic, since to conceive of a species as having dignity is a rather abstract idea. An alternative position might be to address the concerns about patenting human DNA in the context of a claim that the human species is sacred and that such sanctity should not be compromised. It might be added that the species as it currently exists is unreservedly valuable, perhaps even perfect. Scientifically, of course, this makes little sense. To conceive of the human species as sacred, not needing improvement, and something that ought never be altered does *not* fit with medical research nor with a realistic interpretation of the body and human identity. The claim that the human species can be improved implies that it is in fact flawed. Striving for perfection, then, by patenting and engineering 'better' humans would seem quite desirable.

Of course, there can be no denying that genes, together with the understanding of one's genetic heritage are important. The possibility that individuals might be comprised – at least genetically – in part by a manufacturing company would seem bizarre, and one could imagine the psychological difficulties that could arise for such an individual to have an intimate knowledge of their genotype (Häyry and Lehto, 1998). However, where the technology is employed to improve the standard of living, I would suggest that these psychological concerns are negligible. If the choice is between a life in suffering (or no life at all for that matter) or a life where one's genetic heritage is the product of mother, father, and science, then the latter seems more desirable. Nevertheless, whether patenting simply for enhancement purposes would be desirable is another question, which cannot be pursued further in this chapter.

My conclusion here, then, is that if any claim is to be made about human dignity, then a much richer understanding of this concept is required than Kantian principles can supply. It is necessary to consider a definition that is sympathetic to technologies that might stand to affect the species rather than any single individual. However, whether the patenting of life is actually perceived as compromising one's personal identity is a very different question requiring a quite different perspective. It is my suggestion that such ownership need not pose any serious threat to human identity and individual autonomy. The basis of my argument involves appealing to what precisely is owned where DNA might be patented. I argue that the rejection of patenting human DNA as a challenge to the sanctity of the human species is a product of genetic essentialism. That human DNA might belong to a company within the United States, or to anyone for that matter does not seem, to me, unacceptable in principle. Yet, this does not mean allowing organisations to propagate this ownership to do with it as they wish, nor to monopolise this knowledge and its findings. Neither does owning the patent to human DNA mean that any individual is owned by another. Indeed, the limitation on what is owned remains simply with the matter of genes and this alone, I believe, does not jeopardise any sense of autonomy or identity for an individual.

Note

1   See, for example, Harris, J. (1997, June 19), 'Is Cloning an Attack on Human Dignity?', *Nature*, 387, p.754; Harris, J. (1998a). 'Cloning and Human Dignity', *Cambridge Quarterly of Healthcare Ethics*, 7, pp.163-67; Harris, J. (1998b), *Clones, Genes, and Immortality*, Oxford, Oxford University Press; Harris, J. (1999), 'Clones, Genes, and Human Rights', in J. Burley (ed.), *The Genetic Revolution and Human Rights: The Oxford Amnesty Lectures 1998*, Oxford, Oxford University Press, pp.61-94.

References

Harlow, J. and Gould, M. (1999, October 31), 'Parents target Oxbridge egg donors', *The Sunday Times*, p.12.

Harris, R. (1999). *Ron's Angels*, Hypertext Document: http://www.ronsangels.com [Accessed: January 2000].

Häyry, H. and Lehto, T. (1998), 'Who should know about our genetic make-up and why?', *Proceedings of the 20th World Congress of Philosophy*, Boston, Hypertext Document: http://www.bu.edu/wcp/Papers/Bioe/BioeHay1.htm [Accessed: October 1999].

Holtug, N. (1998), 'Creating and Patenting New Life Forms', in H. Kuhse and P. Singer, *A Companion to Bioethics,* Oxford, Blackwell Publishers Ltd, pp.206-214.

Owen, D. (1995), *Patenting Human Genes*, MRC Technology Transfer Group, Hypertext Document: http://www.nimr.mrc.ac.uk/mhe95/genepat.htm [Accessed: April, 2000].

Reiss, M.J. and Straughan, R. (1996), *Improving Nature?: The Science and Ethics of Genetic Engineering,* Cambridge, Cambridge University Press.

Rifkin, J. (1998), *The Biotech Century: Harnessing the gene and remaking the world,* London, Victor Gollancz.

Terragni, F. (1993), Biotechnology Patents and Ethical Aspects, *Cancer Detection and Prevention*, 17(2), pp.317-321.

Wertz, D.C. (1999, February 1), Patenting DNA: A Primer, *Gene Letter* Hypertext Document published by GeneSage: http://www.genesage.com/professionals/geneletter/archives/dna1.html [Accessed: 18 April, 2000).

Chapter 12

Personal Identity and the Protection of Mankind:
Genetics and Legal Philosophy

Grégoire Kantardjian

In this chapter I discuss whether or not the genetic identity a person inherits is a genuine component of his or her personal identity, as well as what limits should be imposed on the new genetics. What is the role played by genes in the constitution of personal identity? And are geneticists the right people to answer such a question?

The idea of limiting or disqualifying genetics in the determination of personal identity has rarely been contemplated or taken seriously. However, it is far from obvious that science can influence social norms or teach us something about man in society, since being a person or an individual requires much more than a simple genetic structure.

In order to make this clear, I will divide this chapter into three sections. First, I believe it is necessary to remind ourselves that science and law are strictly heterogeneous fields. Indeed, ignoring this leads to the usual mistake which consists in saying that biological discoveries and biotechnological progress require the modification of certain aspects of law concerning the manipulation of the human body. Second, I will try to show that the concept of the genetic heritage of mankind is not enough to the protect the human species against the new biotechnological threats. Finally I will propose a new legal conception of the body which could help to protect the individual's integrity and preserve the definition of a human being as we know it.

1. The disqualification of science in the determination of legality

Let me remind my readers of one simple but important point: scientific laws and juridical laws are different in nature and function. The former deal with the world of *natural phenomena*, their function is to cover reality and help man to orientate himself among phenomena. In contrast, the latter deal with *human action*, and their function is to guide action and indicate the limits within which this action must remain.

We must then start by correcting some wrong and unproven opinions about the relationship between science and law. The main *doxa* can be expressed as follows: law has to conform to facts. In the field of biomedical technologies, this opinion can be translated like this: the progress of the biomedical sciences has engendered new possibilities that the ancient law could not contemplate. Therefore, legal systems must now be modified so as to create categories that acknowledge these new scientific discoveries (e.g. the possibility for a widow to bear a child from her deceased husband). Judicial fiction (for indeed, legal categories are fictions) should yield to biological reality. This is what a French jurist calls 'the myth of the coincidence between the objectives of science and human rights' (Labrusse-Riou, 1989), as if scientific progress went along with the improvement of human dignity. This *doxa* ignores several very important issues.

First, science and law do not have the same object. Biology studies the human being as an object, whereas law treats it as a subject. This difference cross-checks with that between reality and fiction, or nature and culture. The content of law is totally independent of scientific discoveries or observations. One reason for this is that science and technology do not convey any conception of man as person and of humankind as a community; they only consider it in its material and mechanical dimension. The very existence of law, however, implies that there is a conviction that a human being is something more than sheer animality and materiality, that humankind is defined by a fundamental absence of determination which is illustrated by its ability to do good or harm. Science and law belong to heterogeneous fields, namely what the Germans call *Sein* and *Sollen*, 'what is' vs. 'what ought to be', reality vs. norm. British readers will be familiar, too, with David Hume's idea that 'is' cannot entail 'ought'. Hume's opinion, indeed, was that no moral conclusion or value judgement could be derived from cognitive propositions. Cognitive propositions are statements about facts, about what is or is not the case, whereas moral judgements are statements about what ought to be. Scientific knowledge, empirical observations are of no help when it comes to normative thought, whether ethical or juridical.

We must also draw a clear distinction between ethics and deontology. Deontology is a code of conduct a group of people with common interests gives to itself. It has nothing to do with rules that must be followed by the entire population, regardless of social and professional position, for the sake of man's dignity and integrity. One major mistake is to accept that deontological (instead of ethical) rules be elevated to the status of legal rules. That is what happened in France in 1994.

The debates on bioethics in France in the 1990s have opposed those who wanted a simple set of rules for genetic manipulations and prenatal selection, and those who asked that the French law included the banning of such manipulations as well as strict control of every biotechnological practice. The French parliament has voted in favour of the first solution, supported by scientists and doctors and supposedly by the French population (which has never been consulted on such a major issue). The way this problem has been resolved has dramatic consequences: French legislation establishes and legalises a separation between body and mind, person and citizen (i.e. legal subject) as well as the ideology of the body seen as something purely material that can be dissected, the organs being like spare parts.

Science and law do not study humans under the same dimension. The essential property of human beings according to biology is life, whereas according to law it is dignity, because dignity encapsulates both the singularity of every being and their membership of the same community of persons. The essence of person is his dignity, which remains unaltered from time immemorial and to all eternity. There is no evolution of dignity, only of the actual enforcement of it through better political systems. The main legal concept concerning the human person is the *unavailability* of the body (which explains why slavery and torture are banned), since hurting the body is not different from hurting the soul and the very essence of the person. Slavery and torture would never have been the objects of moral reprobation and of legal interdiction if people did not have the conviction that, through the body, it is the very dignity of the individual that is denied. In contrast, science, especially biology, does (and has to) consider the body regardless of the soul (or whatever designates the essence and dignity of the person).

One example illustrates this incommensurability of biology and law: that of the so-called 'progressive ontology of the embryo'. The actual data of science seem to indicate that until the 14th day after conception, the embryo as a singular, idiosyncratic person does not yet exist, since it is only a cluster of totipotent cells. It would become *progressively* human. Law, on the other hand, cannot admit that there are degrees of personhood, that one can be a little more of a person or a little less of a holder of right depending on the number of weeks or months of existence, whether it be before or after birth. If law were to be guided by biology, it could only give the embryo the status of a thing (and therefore not a of holder of rights), and the problem would be how to explain that the same 'object' can change from thing to person a certain moment of time. However, French legislation has actually ratified this nonsense by dividing pregnancy into three periods. From conception till the end of the tenth week, the embryo *belongs* to the mother alone, who has a right to get rid of it. This means that the foetus has the status of a thing (it *belongs* to someone - as opposed to any human person, who cannot belong to anyone - and it can be destroyed without legal sanctions). From the tenth week till the sixth month, the foetus is said to be 'not viable'. It has relative protection since abortion can only take place for therapeutic reasons. Finally, after six months, the foetus is said 'viable' and possesses the status of a holder of right and it can be attacked only if the mother's life is in danger.[1] This conception is inspired by biological time, where the foetus becomes only progressively human. In order to avoid a shocking word ('thing') as well as the miraculous transformation of a thing into a person, people use words or expressions such as 'foetus', 'embryo', 'parental project', even 'human material'. This is only a way to hide the problem, which is: how can we rationally justify that some entity does not have the same status nine weeks after the beginning of its existence than six months later on? That the central nervous system, for instance, develops after a certain number of weeks or days or months should be totally irrelevant to law, because being a person has nothing to do with having specific physiological capacities, however important these may be, as is clearly shown by the fact that people in a coma are not deprived of their fundamental rights.

Given that science and law are incommensurable, one can doubt that biology or genetics should be entitled to influence the decisions that societies make about what is allowed and what is not. That is why entrusting advisory committees with a majority of doctors and scientists with the job of making recommendations on bioethical issues makes little sense.

2. The limits of the concept of genetic heritage of mankind

Even though science and law are and must remain independent activities, it is necessary to rethink some aspects of law in the light of new bioethical problems such as prenatal diagnosis and selection, artificial procreation, donation of organs etc. All these practices, due to biomedical progress, raise new threats on the very concept and reality of mankind. The menace of the concrete and symbolic destruction of humankind as we know it induces the demand that its protection be legally guaranteed.

The biotechnological revolution threatens humans directly. This is something we must be aware of. Selecting the sex of children, modifying one's genetic structure in order to eliminate illnesses, manipulating genes, are acts that will have consequences that we cannot predict, especially in the long term. Till now, mankind has never been structurally modified. We have inherited a structure that has remained the same for millions of years. I cannot see what entitles us to modify anything drastically. What we must transmit to future generations is our human identity as we have received it from our ancestors. Twenty years ago, the German philosopher Hans Jonas, in his famous book *The Principal Responsibility*, warned us against the new power we have on the future of our species. This power brings new responsibilities and obligations. Since we are now in a position to modify dramatically our environment, so that future life on earth could become impossible, we must create a new concept of responsibility which makes us responsible not only for what has been done, but also for what will be done. For future generations, although not existent, already have rights today, and we have duties towards them, especially that of preserving the possibility of life on this planet in the distant future. Jonas was one of the first to insist on the fact that being able to do something does not entail that one should do it (something that people always tend to forget). In other words, one cannot conclude from the fact that we can modify genes that we have the right to do this. Whenever the effects of some new invention cannot be predicted, the precautionary principle should prevail.

The ability to change mankind and abolish fate, through prenatal selection for instance, entails new obligations. We cannot take the risk of producing another kind of human being, nor have the arrogance to decide to impose this new definition of a human being on future generations. (We must be all the more cautious in that a philosopher like Peter Sloterdijk has recently evoked the possibility of modifying the human species in order to tame its destructive instincts and reach a new and better level of humanity.)

What, then, can we propose to defend and protect mankind against the new Frankensteins? The global solution is to propose that humanity as a whole be given the status of a holder, or subject, of rights. Since, as the French philosopher Montaigne put it, 'every man carries within himself the entire shape of the human condition', we have to institute some principle which would protect mankind in the very flesh of every individual. The idea is to 'go beyond a conception of law centred on the person taken individually and reach a wider comprehension where mankind is contemplated as the holder of right par excellence' (Terré, 1987).

The only serious proposition has been that made by Jacques Attali (1988), a French author, and A. C. Kiss (1983), a teacher at the Academy of International Rights in the Hague. These authors suggest that human genetic resources be part of the common heritage of mankind, along with extra atmospheric space and the oceans. Attali, for instance, states that 'the material elements of life, such as the embryo or genes, must be given the status of indefeasible properties of the human species, and treated like absolute sanctuaries that cannot be manipulated by man, even if that implies a refusal to treat or correct some genetic defect'.

The main purpose would be to conserve genetic diversity. This technical solution aims at preventing the human genome - which is the material basis of human identity - from being appropriated by any individual, state, organisation, research laboratory or company. Human genetic resources should then be considered as what in Latin was called *res communes*, i.e. common things, things shared in common that no one can appropriate for himself. I see important limits to this approach. First, this would mean gathering all the individual genotypes, a collectivisation incompatible with the defence of the individual as such. This solution entails the depersonalisation of man: in order to protect mankind as a whole, the person disappears into the background; this transfer gives to one side what it takes from the other side, i.e. effective protection, as if it were impossible to protect with equal efficiency humanity and the individuals who embody it. Considering all the individual genetic structures as a whole is incompatible with the singularity involved in the concept of person. Moreover, this idea tends to identify humanity with its genetic structure, while humanity exceeds by far its purely material dimension.

Finally, this approach is too utilitarian to guarantee the protection of human dignity. This management-type attitude ignores the symbolic dimension that *also has to be preserved*, because preserving genetic diversity is absolutely useless if humanity under its cultural and ideal dimension is not preserved as well. Here too much pragmatism could blur the image of what is really at stake with the development of biomedical technologies. The risk with too much emphasis on the genetic aspect of the problem is to forget that genes alone are not enough to create and therefore preserve humanity.

3. A new legal status for the human body

The genetic structure is something we inherit. It is the material element that makes us a species and that makes us individuals. Genetic structure is, like as the idea of humanity, the common ground on which individuation is possible. Furthermore, genes confirm the ancient and mediaeval idea of individuation through matter. They are the material elements which constitute the human species as well as what makes an individual what it is, i.e. the encounter between two genetic programs each of which is the result of a previous encounter, and so on.

But 'individual' does not mean 'person'. Being a person requires more. It is a relational, not a substantial property. It requires belonging to a culture, interacting with other people. It has to do with social exchanges and interactions. It is of no use focussing on genes if one wants to strengthen the protection of humanity. We now have to consider the body on a more general level and analyse the relationship between the body and the subject.

Genes are something we inherit, the body is not something that we possess. This is where Latin law and mediaeval philosophy can give us conceptual instruments to address the new challenges resulting from the recent developments of biotechnology. I suggest, as a means of setting up a judicial status to guard against the alteration of human dignity, to apply to the body the juridical category of usufruct. The body, especially its genetic structure, should be considered not as a possession but as a tenure. This idea is an updating of the ancient distinction between the *usus* and the *abusus*, the former being the right to use a thing, the latter the right to alienate it. This usually applies to houses and apartments. I propose to apply it to the body. Not having the proprietorship over one's own body implies that no alteration of it (all the more reason no genetic modification) is possible, even when one gives one's consent. On the contrary, the people who have the usufruct have the duty to prevent the object from being damaged. The 'object' here is the matter, i.e. the body, which allows the idea of humanity to become concrete, to be embodied. My idea is that every person, through his body, incarnates humanity, so that every body (in the double meaning) must be protected since all damage inflicted on it is a crime against humanity. The best way to protect mankind is, then, to consider that the body is not something we possess, so that we cannot do anything we want with it.

But if the individuals do not own their bodies, who does? A.C. Kiss and the French philosopher Michel Serres (1990) suggest that a number of people (politicians, jurists and scientists) or institutions have to be entrusted with the right to represent humanity (Kiss) or nature (Serres). Such trustees would have the duty to represent the interests of humanity or nature. This idea seems quite reasonable, but it lacks transcendence.

St Thomas Aquinas,[2] in the *Summa Theologica*, writes that man does not have the mastery (*dominium*) over material things, because only God has this *dominium*. Man is not the master or proprietor of nature, God is. Man only possesses the use (*usus*) over material things, and only as far as he wants to do good. If man does not use things with a view to the Good, he cannot claim his right to use those things. This seems a good idea, no matter what name one wants to give to this transcendence (God, Nature, Humanity...). Men have the right to use their bodies and the duty to respect them; some people could be entrusted with the right to sanction any abuse; but mastery over the body should be forever out of reach.

To conclude, I would recall a distinction made within German phenomenology between *Körper* (body) and *Leib* (flesh). The body is the material dimension of the person, whereas 'flesh' designates the singularity of the person who incarnates the body. Flesh is more than sheer materiality; it is the body plus the personal history of the person integrated in his or her body. It seems to me that we can neither possess the body (because we have no right over matter) nor possess flesh (because flesh is inseparable from us, so that there is no minimal distance which could make possession possible). Thus there is no way that the manipulation of genes and the alteration of the human body could be justified or excused.

All this may seem a little bit brutal or extreme, but it has to be such both because of the importance of what is at stake here and because today's blind confidence in the progress of science and technology could turn into a final nightmare.

Notes

1   See B. Edelman (1988), 'Entre personne humaine et matériau humain: le sujet de droit', in Edelman and Hermitte (eds), *L'homme, la nature et le droit*, Paris, C. Bourgois.
2   IIa-IIae, q. 66, a. 1.

References

Attali, J. (1988), *Au propre et au figuré,* Paris, Fayard.
Kiss, A.C. (1983), 'La notion de patrimoine commun de l'humanité', Recueil Cours de la Haye, t. 175.
Labrusse-Riou, C. (1989), 'L'homme à vif: biotechnologies et droits de l'homme', in *Esprit,* Nov. 1989, pp.60-70.
Serres, M. (1990), *Le contrat naturel,* Paris, Flammarion.
Terré, F. (1987), *L'enfant de l'esclave,* Paris, Flammarion, p.210.

PART 3

Genes and the Non-Human World

Chapter 13

Commodifying Animals: Ethical Issues in Genetic Engineering of Animals[1]

Brenda Almond

As previous contributors to this volume have argued, developments in genetic engineering may produce unanticipated consequences. In Parts 1 and 2, the emphasis has been on the implications of this for human-beings. Part 3 takes account of the possible consequences for the non-human world, and for the environment. In all cases, though, there is the possibility that some of these developments may prove impossible to retreat from or to control. Evaluation of the risks is a matter for empirical assessment but there are also considerations which are more specifically ethical. Many of these developments have already been the subject of ethical debate and discussion, but this chapter is limited to discussion of the narrower issue of genetic engineering and consequent patenting of results in the case of non-human living beings.

The question of how humans should behave in relation to non-human animals has been widely discussed by contemporary philosophers (Singer, 1989; Clarke, 1977; Midgley, 1984). Mostly, though, this discussion has focussed on the issue of how we humans treat *individual* animals, whether the debate is about animal experimentation or farming practices. The question is often posed as whether we are free to exploit animals for our own purposes or whether we have a duty of stewardship towards them which includes what we humans like to call humane treatment, as well as a degree of respect for their nature. The answer may depend to some extent on whether we follow Cartesian dualism and see animals as machines, or whether we see them as lesser but broadly similar creatures to ourselves, occupying a place in the great continuum of living beings, and capable of having goals and instincts we can understand and with which we can empathise.

Today, though, another issue is coming to the fore. This is the question of how, in our scientific practices, we treat animal *species* now that new developments in biotechnology have made possible not only genetic modification of whole types - individuals and their offspring in perpetuity - but also creative constructs with no easily recognised forebears. Of course, it could be said that the manipulation of species is not a new issue, since there have been centuries of deliberate cross-breeding of both plants and animals in order to produce animal types more suited to human purposes, from the terrier bred to go down holes in pursuit of rabbits to the sheep favoured for its shaggy wool. But while humans have indeed sought to alter types in this way, it would seem that the sheer acceleration of the pace of change made possible by modern technology means that we are confronting a difference in degree that has become in effect a difference in kind. So the genetic engineering issue must be distinguished from more general questions familiar from debates about animal experimentation or the raising of animals for food.

First, however, it should be said that genetic engineering is a complex, costly and sophisticated scientific process, and so it is hardly surprising that when important innovations in this area have been developed by scientists working for commercial concerns, the businesses involved should try to secure for themselves the profits arising from the new discoveries. Nor is it surprising that they should seek to do this by applying to their inventions existing laws, in particular the law of patents, which were in fact devised to protect inanimate inventions and products, even though in this case, the inventions concerned are living beings.

However, the idea of patenting life raises immediate ethical questions; and objections to the new technology of genetic modification have come from many quarters, not only from well-known or regular advocates of animal rights. Probably the most pervasive charge is that genetic engineering involves what in the past might have been described as 'playing God' but is more likely these days, to be deplored as rashly following Frankenstein. But before discussing these charges, it would be useful first to give one or two examples of the practical possibilities.

The two main fields in which research of this kind is conducted are biomedicine and food production, the latter including both plants and animals. Perhaps the best known development in the biomedical area is the onco-mouse - a mouse bred to be particularly susceptible to cancer, and therefore useful for laboratory investigation in the field of cancer research. In contrast, while the goal of medical research may be to produce animals with *adverse* characteristics, which can effectively model human diseases, the goal of research in the field of animal husbandry is more likely to be the exaggeration of *desired* characteristics. This has already resulted in, for example, a turkey whose breast is so developed that it cannot maintain its balance, and can only reproduce by artificial insemination. Also on the horizon, or possibly already existing in research establishments somewhere in the world, are anencephalic (and therefore insentient) cows and pigs - creatures which occupy a bleak borderland between animal and vegetable.

Various objections are raised to these developments, some of them as much aesthetic as ethical, but before discussing these, it will be useful to set out briefly some of the background to these developments.

Background and context

In 1971, a General Electric microbiologist applied to the US Patent and Trademark Office (PTO) to patent a genetically engineered oil-eating microbe that could be used to clean up oil-spills in the ocean. Now patents, or intellectual property rights, allow their owner to make, use, or sell the product in question, and are granted in the US subject to three criteria: they must be novel; they must be non-obvious; and they must be useful. The GE application was at first rejected by the PTO on the grounds that microbes were 'products of nature' and hence not novel, and also because it was held that life-forms were non-patentable. This position was later reversed when an appeal court ruled that the fact that microbes were animate beings was irrelevant. The Supreme Court later (in 1980) upheld this view, saying that genetically altered organisms could qualify for patent as a new 'manufacture' or 'composition of matter' (Diamond v. Chakrabarty 447 U.S. 303 (1980)).

In 1987, the PTO formally declared that it considered nonnaturally occurring nonhuman multicellular living organisms, including animals, to be patentable subject matter and the following year it approved the oncomouse - the transgenically developed mouse already mentioned which was bred for susceptibility to cancer. It is to be noted that the US Patent Office is not asked to consider ethical aspects of patent applications - something to which an American engineer Chet Fleming deliberately drew attention by applying for and receiving a patent for his 'discorporation' life-support system (never actually used), which was designed to keep the severed head of an animal alive (Fox, 1992, p.137).

The patenting issue was also debated in Europe, starting from a position in the early seventies when, according to the European Patent Convention (EPC), animals were excluded from the scope of patenting law on the grounds that essentially biological processes cannot be patented, although it was permissible to patent microorganisms and microbiological processes. Nevertheless, in 1991, the European Patent Office granted a patent to the oncomouse, believing that the importance of its role in researching cancer treatment outweighed such reservations. Arguing that the oncomouse is not an animal variety but is the result of a microbiological process, the EPO concluded that genetically engineered animals such as the oncomouse could be patented as 'self-replicable matter'. Currently, a draft directive which contrasts significantly with the older European Patent Convention and is intended to enable European firms to compete with US and Japanese companies in a lucrative biotechnology market, would allow patenting of 'biotechnological inventions'. In contrast to these moves, there have been calls from some animal rights activists to redraft the Treaty of Rome to reclassify animals as sentient beings and not as agricultural products or goods.

The present situation is that, despite controversy, an estimated ten thousand or more strains of transgenic mice have now been produced, as well as genetically modified rats, rabbits, sheep, cattle, pigs, poultry and fish. These animals have uses in developmental biology, immunological research, cancer research, and in investigating somatic gene therapy. Animals are also genetically engineered to secrete valuable biologically active compounds for pharmaceuticals in milk, blood, or tissue. In some cases, to achieve compatibility with human recipients, human genetic material is mixed with that of other species. This kind of research has been jokingly referred to as 'molecular pharming'. More conventional farming, however, is also an area of research, with the cloning of prized farm animals a highly publicised priority.

The ethical debate

Many animal welfare organisations have expressed opposition to these developments, as have some agricultural organisations, environmental groups like Friends of the Earth and other public interest organisations including medical groups such as the U.S.-based Physicians' Committee for Responsible Medicine (Fox, 1992, pp.186-87). Adverse reaction has come, too, from religious leaders, some of whom attended a conference in Washington DC in May 1995 which was partly, at least, inspired by the author Jeremy Rifkin's appeal for the 'resacrilization of nature' (Rifkin, 1985). The conference issued an appeal against the patenting of life forms, both human and animal, declaring that '... humans and animals are creations of God, not humans, and as such should not be patented as human inventions' (Peters, 1997, pp.115-26).

Behind such assertions lies the thought that humans may finally have over-stepped the mark in their scientific activities. Both theologians and environmental philosophers are to be found who agree in seeing ventures which involve juggling the very building-blocks of life as a sign of human arrogance - the term often used is the Greek word *hubris*, a word which has no exact equivalent in the English language, but which implies that humans are usurping the prerogatives of the gods. The view is also commonly expressed that genetic engineering of animals violates the dignity and integrity of non-human species.

It is, of course, true that the crossing of species and the creation of new forms of life seems to set humans a god-like challenge. But as has already been pointed out, humans have always interfered with nature, crossing plant and animal species for their own purposes. Nature, however, has usually kept such ventures in check by rendering the product of such manipulation infertile. It is also the case that these processes in animal and plant husbandry have taken place over hundreds of years - slow and largely benign developments which have allowed nature itself its evolutionary role of correction of error and preservation of success. Human experimenters, too, have had time to modify and adapt their efforts in the light of experience. Developments in the last couple of decades, in contrast, have proceeded and are proceeding at an accelerated pace - a process the American philosopher Bernard E. Rollin, in his book *The Frankenstein Syndrome: ethical and social issues in the genetic engineering of animals*, calls 'evolution in the fast lane' (Rollin, 1995, p.108).

But objections to genetic engineering are not based solely on the element of unknown longterm risk. Rollin, who nevertheless gives it his qualified support, suggests that part of the opposition to genetic engineering is based on a deeper philosophical objection to the innate reductionism or scientism of defenders of the new scientific technologies. The idea that mind reduces to biology and biology to chemistry, so that in the end life is nothing but the perpetual motion of a shifting chemical brew may be profoundly disturbing to some human sensibilities (Rollin, 1995, pp.24-32).

Faced with such philosophical as well as more specifically ethical objections, sceptics may decide to challenge the assumption that ethics has anything at all to do with science. More particularly, they may argue that the kind of practical questions that arise in the pursuit of scientific enquiries, especially those involving human-animal relationships, require practical rather than ethical answers. They may well point out, too, that ethicists and moral philosophers themselves often seem to offer conflicting perspectives.

In reply to such scepticism, let us admit that ethics do not present just one face - there are a number of approaches to ethics which might superficially appear to lead to different conclusions. I would suggest, however, that this impression is deceptive. For although the main ethical theories start from very different premises, they have in common a willingness to take seriously the issue of human animal relationships - to accept, one way or another, that animals matter morally. Hence there could be said to be, implicitly at least, a degree of consensus amongst theorists about the moral status of animals which is highly relevant to legal moves such as patenting, which treat animals, explicitly or implicitly, as commodities, or things. This claim of a common viewpoint is best explained by looking briefly at some of the main approaches to ethics.

The utilitarian approach

The system of ethics it may seem most natural to appeal to in relation to animal welfare is that of utilitarianism - the theory that makes the maximisation of welfare the standard of right and wrong. But, while many of the most prominent champions of animal welfare are indeed utilitarians, the theory itself is a two-edged sword. For a system of justification that depends in the end on cost-benefit calculation can very easily be used to defend the uncontrolled exploitation of possibilities offered by technological development. For example, it can be used to justify factory-farming practices which ignore the natural instincts of animals in the drive to maximise the production of cheap food. In the recent extreme case of BSE, of course, when grass-eating mammals were made to become cannibalistic carnivores, it turned out that this had the distinctly non-utilitarian outcome of posing a serious threat to human health, as well as devastating economic consequences. But utilitarianism can also - more relevant to the issues to be dealt with here - be used to justify genetic experiments as long as their declared object is to add to human or animal well-being.

So although many leading advocates of animal welfare are utilitarians, it is hard to see that utilitarianism itself directly guarantees animals a parallel place in the same moral universe as human beings. It can only do this indirectly via an independent judgement that animals count - that their happiness and welfare matter. But this is a judgement the grounds for which utilitarianism itself cannot supply. This is why we find utilitarian advocates of animal rights debating, for example, whether even forms of life which threaten human health and welfare must be protected and preserved. The question poses a difficulty for them, simply because to value some sentient beings more than others is to import a notion of value from some quite different source. Nevertheless, the judgement that the happiness or welfare of non-human animals is to be included in utilitarian calculation is one that most utilitarians are inclined to make, taking their inspiration from a famous remark of Jeremy Bentham, utilitarianism's founding father. Opposing those who argued that the intellectual simplicity of animals ruled out consideration of their interests, Bentham wrote: 'The question is not Can they reason? nor Can they talk? but Can they suffer?' (Bentham, 1970. First pub. 1789).

A contemporary defender of Bentham's principle is the utilitarian philosopher Peter Singer, whose book *Animal Liberation*, first published in 1975, is often cited as the start of the contemporary animal rights movement (Singer, 1975). Many people do, however, find it more natural to express their concern for animals in terms of an ethic of rights than an ethic of utility, and this is why utilitarians involved in the animal debate often make common cause with moral philosophers whose arguments are based, not on the welfare principle, but on the central moral notions of rights and justice (Regan and Singer, 1989).

The rights approach

The first thing to notice here is that, like utilitarians, rights theorists, too, must make an independent judgement that animals are to be included in the moral community, and not all of them are willing to do so. One reason is that they fear this may have the effect of diminishing the cause of universal human rights - a cause which is far from having won universal respect or observance as yet. Others, however, see a case for extending recognition at least to those animals that are closest to us biologically. Apes, for example, share more than 98 per cent of our genetic make-up and have many human characteristics and modes of behaviour. Indeed, they are currently the focus of a campaign for parallel recognition, which persuaded the New Zealand government to consider seriously legislating along these lines, although it rejected the proposal in the end. The interests, too, of dogs, cats and horses are regarded as important by many who have learned to appreciate the human-like qualities and intelligence of these 'companion-animals'.

Nevertheless, the claim that animals are moral and legal persons in the same way as humans is too strong for most people. Commonsense would seem to suggest a position somewhere between the view that they are of equal concern and the view that dismisses the interests of non-human animals as negligible. One solution, proposed by the British philosopher Robin Attfield, is to distinguish moral standing from moral significance. It would follow from this that while we can indeed allot moral standing to lesser creatures, we may still legitimately decide to sacrifice them for beings of greater moral significance (Attfield, 1991).

Such a view is consistent with the idea that the relation between human and non-human animals should be one of stewardship rather than exploitation. This notion can claim support from a religious as well as a moral perspective, although this is often overlooked by those who read the creation story in Genesis as giving man dominion over the beasts of the field but fail to read on to discover that even the ox is to be allowed its sabbath day, and worked with care and consideration.

The virtue approach

Perhaps, however, the ethical position that provides the most useful starting-point for consideration of the role and place of animals is neither utilitarianism nor rights theory, but the form of neo-Aristotelianism usually described as virtue ethics (Aristotle, 1976). At first sight, this may seem an unlikely claim, for virtue theory, superficially viewed, is about the cultivation by human beings of specifically human virtues – in classical times courage, temperance, justice, wisdom; faith, hope and charity in the Christian era. In addition, virtue ethics is perhaps best described as the theory which replaces such questions as 'What rules ought we to follow?' or 'What will produce the best results?' with the questions 'How ought I (as an individual) to live?' and 'What is the good society?' (MacIntyre, 1984). To see the relevance of this approach to the issues under discussion here, it is necessary to look behind these questions and see what is the basis for asking them, and what is assumed about how to find answers to them.

Behind the questions, then, and offering an answer to them, is the idea of flourishing. This concept in many ways more useful to those who are seeking an ethic for animal treatment than the cruder measure of utility. The notion of flourishing is fundamentally teleological. It derives from the idea that every kind of object has its own essential end or function. A chair is, for example, not a design object, but something for sitting on. A knife is for cutting, a musical instrument is for making music. The Greek word for excellence, *arete*, is the word we translate as 'virtue'. So the excellence of a chair, a knife, a musical instrument, consists in its being able to fulfil its essential function (*ergon*) well. We might speak of an ideal chair, an ideal knife, etc. with approval. The thought that this generates, then, is that for an object or a creature to flourish, is for it to be in a state or situation that allows it to fulfil its essential function well. As far as human beings are concerned, this may well be a matter of displaying the traditional virtues. More broadly, however, flourishing may be taken as a matter of well-being or health in general, and the flourishing of animals and plants is easily graspable by analogy - the plant which has been left in a dark cellar, for example, metaphorically struggles to find the light it needs to blossom in its appropriate shape and colour - to become what we, as onlookers, know it can be, given the right conditions. Viewed negatively, today's genetic engineering could be said to violate this notion of a final end or goal - a *telos*. On the other hand, of course, viewed positively, it could be said to supply a new human-needs-based *telos*. It is the need to decide between these two perspectives - the negative and the positive - that lies at the heart of the discussion about the creation of life-forms in the laboratory. From the viewpoint of any of the main ethical theories, however, the starting-point for that discussion, can reasonably be the claim that animals matter morally.

The case against genetic engineering of animals

So far the points that have been raised here involve very broad philosophical considerations and, while not disputing their importance, it is clear that there are also arguments - social, environmental, scientific and economic - of a more immediate and practical nature to be considered. These fall into a number of categories.

Safety issues

Perhaps the most obvious area of concern is that developments in genetic engineering may produce effects and consequences that have been unanticipated or overlooked. Some of these may involve harm to humans, e.g. products may be carcinogenic, or they may produce resistance to antibiotics. They may also involve harm to animals, but that issue is best dealt with under a separate heading. Another possibility, a popular subject for fiction-writers, is that undesirable creations could escape by human error, as in the novel *Jurassic Park*. Longterm effects, too, are difficult to predict - abnormalities are to be expected and there is always the fear of developments getting out of hand. Given the ultimate unassessibility of these risks, it is worth noting that public opinion, when consulted, tends to favour safety above economics or even convenience.

But while risk of harm to humans is indeed a valid negative ethical consideration, the judgment that a process or product is safe is not in itself a guarantee of its ethical legitimacy. So, as Rollin writes: 'given the unformed nature of social values regarding genetic engineering and its risks and benefits; given the bad ethical concerns that have replaced good ones; given the definite desire on the part of the public to participate in decision making on genetic engineering; given the fact that people believe that biotechnology will benefit them, yet also are ignorant and fearful of it - all these factors militate in favor of meaningful, serious regulation that addresses these issues, for plainly biotechnology will stand or fall with public acceptance or rejection, not with the progress of the science' (Rollin, 1995, p.102).

Environmental effects

Another source of opposition to genetic engineering comes from a new sensitivity to environmental issues. Sometimes these concerns are dismissed as a form of irrational environmental conservatism that would preserve the natural world just as it is, no matter what. However, environmentalists may have serious and well-supported fears. In particular, they fear a modern enactment of the story of Pandora's box. For once a genetically engineered organism has been released into, or escaped into the environment, it may be impossible to call it back. So predator insects for pest control could themselves become pests, and bigger and more disease-resistant animals may crowd out other animals, leading to the extinction of familiar species which have a vital role in the ecological chain.

There are risks, too, in the loss of genetic diversity. If, for instance, producers decide to settle for agricultural monoculture - drastically reducing, for example, the types of chicken that are bred - a single new disease organism could threaten the survival of the whole species.

Economic aspects

Other objections to the genetic engineering and patenting of animals may be based on the economic consequences of these practices.The narrow profit margins of contemporary agriculture already risk substituting profit for care and also for job satisfaction. Business has squeezed costs in animal agriculture so far that the margin of profit on an individual animal is trivial. This is part of a form of industrialised agriculture based on drugs and chemicals which requires a vast input of energy, generating other environmental problems in the disposal of waste, in ground water contamination and in the many food 'scares' which are a part of modern life.

In these circumstances, further developments involving the genetic modification of farm animals threaten to price out traditional farming altogether, as small family farms find themselves unable to compete with biotechnical agri-business. For the success of traditional farming depends on working in harmony with the natural needs and characterisitcs of animals. Genetic engineeering bypasses such constraints, achieving short-term gains, by strategies which may not be sustainable in the longterm - developing, for example, pigs whose size has been increased by human growth hormone to a size well beyond the natural capacity of land animals.

The objections, however, are not only concerned with cost. As the American writer Michael Fox puts it: 'Subjective economic concerns - which some call greed - should not take precedence over reason, compassion, respect, and justice' (Fox, 1992, p.136). In particular, he suggests, the patenting of animals reflects an exploitative and domineering cultural attitude, which puts human ends above everything else.

Animal welfare issues

When the focus of debate shifts in this way to a conflict of interest between humans and animals, concerns about animal welfare are expressed on two fronts. First, many animal rights activists believe that transgenic research itself involves cruelty to animals; and secondly, they draw attention to the possible suffering of the transgenic animals. The first point raises issues familiar from more general debates about vivisection. These concern the relative claims of animals and humans to moral consideration, the weight of human suffering in comparison to that of animals, and questions about possible absolute limits to what it is legitimate for a human being to do to an animal.

As far as the second charge is concerned, it would be hard to deny that suffering is the lot of laboratory animals which are bred to develop cancer or AIDS.

But agricultural animals, too, may suffer when they are pushed beyond the natural limits of their species - kidney and liver problems, as well as defective joints and limbs, are commonly occurring problems. These are all negative considerations, but, of course, defenders of the new developments put forward a vigorous positive case in response to such objections, and this can be set out in fairly concise terms.

The case *for* research and patenting

It is, of course, to be expected that biotechnology companies and the scientists who work for them should defend the work they are doing. But a number of philosophical commentators, too, have accepted scientific progress in these areas as inevitable and, in many ways, desirable. The heart of their case is that the goals of curing disease and feeding the hungry are beneficent and deserving of ethical respect. Amongst those who offer this defence is Ted Peters who, in his book *Playing God? Genetic determinism and human freedom*, supports the argument of the biotechnology industry that patenting is needed to protect companies' investments in new technologies which have as their end-product therapies for life-threatening disease (Peters, 1997). In addition, he argues that, as far as theological considerations are concerned, creation (in the form of evolution) is ongoing, and that those who talk of God's prerogatives can be reminded that on the whole God leaves improving on nature to human beings. This, at least, is the premiss on which most medicine and medical science is based.

Peters is not alone in arguing that there is nothing sacred about the way nature has presented the world to us and in pointing out that genetic alteration has gone on over thousands of years. Nor is he alone in arguing that as long as safety issues are addressed, and legislation protects animals as far as possible from suffering, it is morally acceptable to proceed with caution. Added to this, it can be argued that there are issues of principle involved: the principle of freedom to conduct scientific research without governmental interference, and the principle of fairness in the allocation of rights to scientific processes: that those who invent highly sophisticated processes deserve to benefit from their skills and labour.

In sum, then, the positive case is first and foremost based on welfare considerations, buttressed and supported by arguments for freedom to pursue scientific research and justice in the allocation of rewards for the fruits of that research.

Finding a balance

The issues, then, are complex and there are weighty considerations on both sides. It may be that no important principles are violated if microbes and viruses, which paved the way for patenting life forms, are legally regarded as patentable items and, indeed, the non-scientific observer may feel more secure if there are controls in this area. But mammals are a different matter, and once transgenic animals exist, they are not *things*. They deserve protection as living and pain-sensitive creatures.

Nevertheless, it may be difficult to explain or to justify the moral unease generated by the deliberate bringing into being of creatures like the oncomouse or the AIDS mouse, which are bred to disease. Here the Arisotelian ideal of the flourishing of a type or species may hold the key. For if we seek objective scientific criteria for flourishing, these can be found in the case of both animals and humans in i) life-span survival and ii) ability to reproduce unaided. Applying these criteria can provide a *prima facie* objection to the creation of disease-model animals, as well as to some genetic modifications of farm animals, which is at the same time both rational and ethical. Laboratory animals often violate the first of these criteria, and many agro-products violate the second. It is a further consideration that the latter tend to be dependent on drugs and interventions throughout their lifespan. In contrast, the guiding principles from an environmental point of view, in agriculture in general, not only in the organic movement, are sustainability and less reliance on chemicals.

It may be argued, however, that medical progress would be restricted by a complete ban on the genetic engineering of laboratory animals and the possibility of patenting the results of research. In reply to this objection, it is worth pointing out that public health and hygiene measures probably play a larger role in the health improvement of the population as a whole than does animal experimentation. Nevertheless, it has to be admitted that an end to experimentation on animals can hardly be expected in the foreseeable future. It may be better in the meantime, therefore, simply to insist, as most developed countries do, on laws to protect animals from suffering, such as enforcing the use of anaesthetics, tranquillisers and analgesics and on euthanasia without a return to consciousness. End-points such as tumour size could also be agreed and multiple surgical use of the same animal banned. Similarly sensitive rules could and should be drawn up in relation to farm animals, although at present these have less protection than laboratory animals.

So what is to be said to those who argue for complete deregulation on free market principles? Well, first it must be said that when ethics and economics appear to conflict, the picture is not always as straightforward as it seems. For market freedom is part of a liberal philosophical position, itself morally based, which includes as a principle the protection of the vulnerable. Once again, then, the issue turns, first of all, on agreeing the status of animals rather than on any empirical calculations. But it also involves an appraisal of the future harm claim, since anything which threatens the life or health of individuals is a legitimate matter for control, even from a libertarian perspective. It is not a violation of free trade and libertarian principles, then, to seek to control some of these developments in biotechnology, not only for the sake of the animals themselves, but also in the public interest and in order to preserve for future generations a heritage which includes important species that we, in the present generation, hold in trust for them. The *loss* of species represents an infringement of the liberty of choice of these future people, and there is no reason why libertarian concern should stop with the present.

We are poised, then, between a vision of unlimited promise and the incalculable threat of the unknown. Some of the things we are doing are, by strict ethical standards, wrong, and ideally would be abandoned. However, it is not possible to be wholly against modern technology, not only because we value its success as a contribution to our way of life, but also because we can be sure that secret laboratories elsewhere in the world will pursue technology to its limits. It may be best, then, to aim for sensible regulation, caution, and protecting what we have. Rollin sums up many of these requirements as 'respect for animals, humans, nature and risk' (Rollin, 1995, p.214).

A final thought

In the book of Genesis, a picture is painted of God creating animals for human use, but requiring them to be treated with care and respect. The story of Noah adds an image of the animals entering the Ark two by two - the natural self-prolongation of species. These images are deeply ingrained in the mind of western human beings. A modern biotechnology company will perhaps shrug off mention of ancient myths, but this would be foolish - myth and culture are what make up our identity and our civilisation. We throw them over at our peril, especially if we are doing it in the name of making a better world.

Note

1   This chapter is substantially based on my article 'Commodifying Animals: ethical issues in the genetic engineering of animals' which was published in the journal Health, Risk and Society, vol.2, 2000 (website http://www.tandf.co.uk). My thanks to the editor and publishers for permission to reproduce this material.

References

Almond, B. (1998), *Exploring Ethics: a traveller's tale*, Oxford, Blackwell.
Aristotle (1976), *Ethics*, trans. J.A.K. Thomson, rev. H. Tredennick, Harmondsworth, Penguin.
Attfield, R. (1991), *The Ethics of Environmental Concern*, 2nd edn., Athens, GA, and London, University of Georgia Press.
Bentham, J. (1970), *An Introduction to the Principles of Morals and Legislation* London, Athlone Press, first published 1789.
Clark, S. (1977) *The Moral Status of Animals*, Oxford, Oxford University Press.
Diamond v. Chakrabarty 447 U.S. 303 (1980).
Fox, Michael W. (1992), *Superpigs and Wondercorn: the brave new world of technology and where it may lead*, New York, Lyons and Burford.
Macintyre, A. (1981), *After Virtue*, London, Duckworth. 2nd edn., 1984.
Midgley, M. (1984), *Animals and Why they Matter*, Harmondsworth, Penguin.

Peters, T. (1997), *Playing God? Genetic determinism and human freedom*, London, Routledge.

Regan, T and P. Singer (eds) (1989), *Animal Rights and Human Obligations*, 2nd edn., Englewood Cliffs, NJ: Prentice-Hall.

Rifkin, J. (1985), *Declaration of a Heretic,* Boston, Routledge and Kegan Paul.

Rollin, Bernard E. (1995), *The Frankenstein Syndrome: ethical and social issues in the genetic engineering of animals*, Cambridge, Cambridge University Press.

Singer, P. (1990), *Animal Rights*, 2nd edn., New York, Random House, first pub. 1975.

Chapter 14

Genetically Modified Crops and the Precautionary Principle: Is There a Case for a Moratorium?

Jonathan Hughes

Introduction

In Britain and many other countries the introduction of genetically modified crops (GM) has become a matter of intense political controversy. Environmental pressure groups such as Friends of the Earth and Greenpeace have played a leading role in opposing GM crops, and have joined with many others in demanding a moratorium on their use. The present chapter offers an assessment and critique of the environmental case for a moratorium as articulated by such groups. In focusing on the environmental case I am not denying the significance of other considerations such as food safety and consumer choice, but rather acknowledging that these are separate issues which need to be assessed independently of one another. Although the issues of food and environmental safety have often been run together in the public debate, not least by those campaigning against GM crops, they are in fact distinct in practice as well as in theory. This can be seen by considering that GM foods produced in contained factory conditions would pose little or no threat to the environment, while GM crops such as cotton or industrial oilseed rape raise questions about environmental impact but not about food safety. In focusing on the environmental impact of GM crops, therefore, I am simply setting aside the other issues for separate consideration.

The view taken in this chapter is that while some of the environmental risks highlighted by opponents of GM crops are real and potentially serious, they do not justify the demand for a blanket moratorium. This matters for several reasons. Firstly, an unjustified moratorium would mean that the potential benefits of the technology would be unwarrantedly foregone, and this could be unjust to potential beneficiaries of the technology. In making this point, the Nuffield Council's report on GM crops[1] focuses in particular the apparent injustice of depriving the world's poor of the opportunity to benefit from the increased food supply and employment that might result from the development of new high-yielding crop varieties. Other potential benefits of importance to the least advantaged in our global society include the development of crops with enhanced nutritional content (e.g. vitamin A enriched rice to combat the deficiency which often leads to blindness in regions where rice is the staple food), crops engineered to provide vaccination against common diseases, and crops tolerant of particular growing conditions such as drought and soil acidity. Secondly, foregoing the benefits of GM crops could be counterproductive from an environmentalist perspective, resulting in the loss of opportunities to reduce the environmental damage associated with conventional agriculture. It has been claimed, for example, that GM crops can reduce the need for chemical inputs such as pesticides, herbicides and fertilisers, and can ease soil erosion and moisture loss in vulnerable areas by eliminating the need for ploughing.[2] Whether or not the particular claims made for current GM crops are true there seems to be no reason in principle why GM crops should not produce benefits as well as risks for the environment. Thirdly, the demand for a moratorium could be a *political* mistake for environmentalists. Indiscriminate opposition to GM crops may give ammunition to those who would write off *all* opposition to biotechnology as Luddite, undermining the ability of environmentalists to object effectively to particular technologies as well as diminishing more generally the authority with which their views are received by the public.

This chapter begins by categorising and appraising the possible grounds for a moratorium. It then considers the so-called 'Precautionary Principle', arguing that only an unacceptably strong interpretation of the principle would justify a strict moratorium. Finally, it concludes that the arguments point towards a regulatory regime which does not discriminate in principle between GM and other new crop varieties, which evaluates all new crops on a case-by-case basis, and which balances risks against benefits rather than attempting to eliminate them altogether.

Intrinsic grounds for a moratorium

Objections to the use of GM crops may be intrinsic or extrinsic. Intrinsic objections hold that the use of GM crops (or some necessary aspect of their use) is wrong in itself, while extrinsic (or instrumental) objections hold that their use is wrong because of its likely consequences.

The clearest intrinsic objection holds that the *process of genetic modification* itself is morally wrong. This, however, needs clarification. It is often pointed out that humans have been engaged in forms of genetic modification since the dawn of agriculture, by selective breeding and by altering the environment within which natural selection takes place. What is distinctive about the so-called GM crops is not the fact of genetic modification, but the means (and consequently also the speed and extent) of its achievement. Opponents of GM crops typically argue against the thesis that genetic engineering is simply an extension of traditional plant breeding by pointing to the ability of the former to transfer genes between different and highly dissimilar species.[3] We can therefore take this to be the focus of the intrinsic objection. But, while some opponents of GM crops subscribe to such an objection (often characterising the transfer of genes across species boundaries as 'playing God' or 'interfering with nature'[4]), this view has played little explicit role in the public debate. Indeed, some of the leading opponents of GM crops have taken care to dissociate themselves from such a view by approving the use of GM technology under contained conditions, for example for medical purposes.[5] In my view they are right to do so, since I can see no reason why gene transfer should be held immoral while selective breeding – which may equally be guided by genetic knowledge and aimed at results that would never occur without human intervention – is not. Given the many and diverse 'interferences with nature' which we not only accept but regard as important steps in the struggle against poverty, disease and the destructiveness of nature, it is not clear what reason we could have for drawing the boundary of permissible interference just short of gene transfer.[6] Moreover, even if the view in question can be given a coherent motivation, it remains a minority view, dependent upon a particular conception of the value of naturalness, and as such cannot be imposed on those who quite reasonably take a different view without violating such liberal canons as neutrality between conceptions of the good, or Mill's Harm Principle.

A view related to the one just described, but which is more properly an environmental objection and may play a more significant role in the controversy about GM crops, asserts the intrinsic badness not of the process of genetic modification itself, but of the *release of genetically modified material into the environment*. It holds that the environment is degraded or devalued by the mere presence of genetically modified material, independently of any perceptible effects. This view is discussed in the Nuffield report, and appears to be a necessary underpinning for the stance of Greenpeace and others that, while contained use of GM organisms (GMOs) is acceptable, the inevitability of genes escaping from GM crops into the wider environment ('genetic pollution') is, independently of any further consequences, sufficient ground for halting their use and engaging in civil disobedience to destroy existing crops.[7]

This view straddles the distinction between intrinsic and extrinsic objections to the use of GM crops. Insofar as the environment that is 'polluted' by GM material is conceived as distinct from the agricultural land on which the crop is planted, the objection is an extrinsic one since the spreading of GM material into the environment will be a consequence rather than a constituent element of its use. However, the fact that this consequence – 'genetic pollution' – is itself seen as intrinsically bad is significant. If the badness of 'genetic pollution' depended upon further consequences (such as loss of biodiversity) which can also arise from other causes, then the consequences of GM agriculture would have to be quantified and weighed against the similar consequences of the alternative agricultural systems that GM agriculture might replace. Holding 'genetic pollution' to be intrinsically bad, by contrast, allows opponents to treat it as uniquely bad and thus to maintain an absolute opposition to GM crop use while accepting the use of GMOs in contained environments.

However, this view faces objections similar to those facing the stronger intrinsic view. Firstly, it is hard to see how the mere presence of modified genetic material in an ecosystem can constitute a significant disvalue, given that the areas most likely to be affected by agricultural biotechnology already bear the heavy imprint of conventional agriculture and other human activities. And secondly, this view, like the previous one, rests on a particular conception of the value of 'naturalness' which cannot justify unlimited restrictions on those who quite reasonably do not share it. In the absence of consensus, then, the most that can be justified by this view (or rather by the interests of those who hold it) would appear to be the maintenance of GM-free buffer zones to protect particular areas of relative wilderness from genetic 'pollution'.

Extrinsic grounds for a moratorium

Let us now turn our attention to the extrinsic grounds for a moratorium, which have featured more prominently in the public debate over GM crops and are more central to the environmentalist agenda. In discussing these I take as my source a report by Friends of the Earth which calls for a 5-year moratorium on the commercial growing, testing and marketing of GM seeds and foods, and cites (with reference to the scientific literature) fourteen possible effects of GM crops which it takes to comprise the 'scientific basis' for such a moratorium.[8] The possible effects cited are as follows (the numbering is mine but otherwise the points are as they appear in the report's summary and section 3):

1   Transgenic inserts into crops may be unstable.
2   Genes from GM crops will be transferred by pollen to wild relatives and non GM crops.
3   GM traits are likely to be incorporated into populations of the wild relatives of oilseed rape and sugar beet.
4   Transgenes could be transferred from GM crops to soil bacteria.
5   Horizontal transfer may already have occurred at test sites.
6   Herbicide tolerant corps may seriously threaten biodiversity in agricultural areas.
7   Widespread use of glufosinate and glyphosate could affect soil ecosystems and so affect crop performance and nutrient cycling.
8   Herbicide tolerant volunteers may become established in crop rotations leading to weed control problems and further applications of herbicide.
9   Insect pests may rapidly develop resistance to GM crops expressing Bt toxins, shortening the useful life of such crops and compromising the effectiveness of existing Bt insecticides.
10 Pest resistant crops may have adverse impacts on beneficial insects and other invertebrate populations.
11 It will be impossible to ensure that GM foods will not cause new allergies.
12 GM crops expressing proteins toxic to pests may also be toxic to humans.
13 Exposure to glufosinate and glyphosate residues for both humans and animals is likely to increase with the introduction of herbicide tolerant crops.
14 Antibiotic resistance could be passed onto pathogens and lessen the effectiveness of important drugs.

The first thing to note about this list is that, with the exception of point 2, what is being claimed is that certain effects *may* or *could* ensue, or cannot be guaranteed not to ensue. We are dealing therefore with risk rather than certainty. Moreover, no attempt is made to quantify the risk; the nearest the list comes to a quantification is in 3, where an effect is described as 'likely'. Secondly, not all of the effects listed are relevant to the concerns of this paper. 11-14 are matters of food safety and medical, rather than environmental, concern, and will therefore not be discussed further (although some of the points made below are in fact applicable to them). Thirdly, 3 is an instance of 2, and 5 is an instance of 4. This leaves 1, 2, 4, 6, 7, 8, 9 and 10 as the potential risk types to be considered. These may be grouped into four categories: *risks associated with herbicide tolerance* (6, 7 and 8), *risks associated with pest resistance* (9 and 10), *risks from gene transfer* (2 and 4), and *risks from crop instability* (1). The remainder of this section will consider each category in turn, giving particular attention to the *scope* of each risk, i.e. the range of crop types to which it applies.

Risks associated with herbicide tolerance

Herbicide tolerant crops (currently the subject of controversial field trials in Britain) are designed to tolerate being sprayed with particular broad spectrum herbicides, which will destroy weeds but leave the crop undamaged. This is claimed to be cheaper and more effective than the alternative of targeting particular weeds with more specific herbicides. Opponents argue, however, that the increased effectiveness of weed control made possible by these crops may threaten biodiversity, causing the decline and disappearance of weed species with similar consequences for invertebrate and bird populations higher up the food chain. It is also claimed that the particular herbicides used with these crops may disrupt soil ecosystems, and that herbicide tolerant 'volunteers' (plants from one year's crop which reappear as weeds in a subsequent year's crop) may cause weed control problems and lead to additional applications of herbicides.

The first thing to note about these risks is that, since they are associated not with GM crops as such but with the specific trait of herbicide tolerance, they cannot justify a blanket prohibition on the use of GM crops. Secondly, the trait of herbicide tolerance is not exclusive to GM crops but has also been produced by conventional selective breeding techniques.[9] The risks associated with herbicide tolerance therefore provide no grounds for singling out GM crops for special regulatory treatment. Any regulatory regime intended to limit these risks should be focused on the '*functional type*' of herbicide tolerant crops rather than the imperfectly correlated '*genetic type*' of GM (transgenic) crops.

The question of whether that regulatory regime should take the form of a moratorium on *herbicide tolerant* crops raises a dilemma. The environmental impact of such crops is a matter of dispute, with supporters claiming that they will *benefit* the environment relative to conventional farming, by allowing the use of less persistent herbicides, by allowing farmers to delay spraying, and perhaps to spray less, and by eliminating the need for ploughing in soils vulnerable to erosion and moisture loss. Both sides claim scientific support, and if scientists really are divided it is hard to see how this dispute can be resolved without fairly extensive field trials involving a variety of crop management practices, environmental conditions and so on. A moratorium which precluded such trials would therefore appear vulnerable to a critique analogous to Mill's critique of censorship. Just as censorship, for Mill, deprives us of the means of establishing the falsity of the censored opinion, so a ban on field trials would deprive us of the means of establishing whether the facts are such as to justify the ban. On the other hand, supporters of a moratorium point out that trials cannot be carried out without creating exposure to the very risks they are intended to assess. Such experimentation is said to involve 'treating the world as a laboratory', and to be in violation of the Precautionary Principle. This principle itself, however, is in need of interpretation and justification, and so we will return to the question of field trials in that context.

Risks associated with pest resistance

The next category of risks relates to pest resistant crops, and my argument here mirrors the one just given. Pest resistant crops secrete substances toxic to the pests that feed on them, but these may also affect non-target organisms, and may lead to a build-up of resistance in the target pest population, compromising the effectiveness both of the crops themselves and of conventionally-applied insecticides, including the Bt insecticide used by organic farmers. However, firstly, these risks are again associated with a functional type (in this case pest resistant crops) rather than with GM crops as such, and so cannot justify a ban on all and only GM crops. And secondly, the extent of these effects, and whether they are greater or less than the effects of conventionally applied insecticides, is disputed, so again we face the choice of trials which create exposure to the risks they are designed to assess, or a moratorium which undermines its own epistemic basis.

Risks from gene transfer

The third set of risks concerns the problem of gene transfer. All kinds of GM crops (except sterile ones) are liable to transfer genes to wild relatives or other crops through wind- or insect-carried pollen, but so too are non-GM crops; so to justify a special regulatory regime it would have to be shown that gene transfer from GM crops is especially damaging. If we discount the intrinsic objection to 'genetic pollution' discussed above, then this would require that some concrete harm be specified beyond the mere presence of genetically modified material in the environment.

The spectre most frequently raised in this context is that herbicide tolerant crops will hybridise with weeds around field margins to create herbicide tolerant 'superweeds'. However, this scenario again relates to herbicide tolerant crops, whether GM or not, rather than to GM crops as such. More generally, hybrids may become 'weedy', and displace their wild relatives – threatening biodiversity and genetic resources – if they acquire some trait that gives them a competitive advantage. This broadens the range of crop varieties that could be problematic, but nevertheless the ability to confer competitive advantage on hybrid offspring will be associated with functional type rather than genetic type: varieties with *environmentally adaptive* modifications such as pest resistance or drought tolerance may well pose a risk, whether produced by GM or not, while those modified in respect of their nutritional or pharmaceutical properties are unlikely to do so. Moreover, the risk of hybridisation depends upon the presence of wild relatives and so applies, for example, to oilseed rape and sugarbeet in Europe, potatoes and maize in South America, but not vice versa.[10] So, once again, the risks do not apply to all and only GM crops, but in this case to particular combinations of functional type and geographical location.

The Friends of the Earth report also cites the 'horizontal transfer' of genes from GM crops to soil bacteria as one of the grounds for a moratorium. The significance of this is that traits could be passed to non-related organisms, negating the last point made above. However, the phenomenon of horizontal transfer is not confined to GM crops, so again this does not provide grounds for discriminating in principle between GM and other novel crop varieties, and again the likely harms would depend on the traits of the crop in question. Moreover, the report indicates no specific consequences likely to result from horizontal transfer. Its suggestion appears to be that this is a source uncertainty and that we should refrain from planting GM crops precisely because we do not know what the consequences might be. It will be argued below, however, that an assertion of risk as lacking in specificity as this (i.e. the mere possibility of as-yet-unidentified bad effects) is insufficient to justify a moratorium.

Risks from crop instability

The final class of risks cited in the Friends of the Earth report is that of crop instability. The report makes the *broad* claim that transgenic inserts may be unstable, and in consequence 'current testing regimes are not always able to predict behaviour of GM crops in the wider environment'. However, the scientific evidence cited relates to the *more specific* claim that transgene inserts may be *deactivated*, or 'silenced' – for example as a consequence of viral infection – leading to the loss of the corresponding traits such as herbicide tolerance. This is a lot less unpredictable. Loss of herbicide tolerance could lead to crop failure following herbicide spraying (and may have done so), but this is more a problem for the farmer than for the environment, and could, at least in developed countries, be adequately addressed by guarantees of compensation from the seed companies. Loss of other traits could be harmful in other ways, but in each case the risk would be specific to the trait in question. Citing crop instability as a ground for a *general* moratorium on GM crops seems to require the stronger claim that *all* GM crops are liable to behave in environmentally damaging ways, but it is not clear that there is any positive evidence for this, and in the absence of such evidence the use of this risk to justify a moratorium must presuppose a strong and contentious version of the Precautionary Principle. It is to this principle that we must now turn.

The Precautionary Principle and the ethics of risk

The Precautionary Principle is usually taken to comprise one or both of the following injunctions:

1   decision-makers should act to protect the environment from harm in advance of scientific certainty about its causes;
2   the burden of proof should be shifted onto the proponent of an activity to show that it is safe before it is permitted.[11]

Claim 1, taken as it stands, seems unexceptionable. In pure scientific research it may be appropriate to demand high (e.g. 95 per cent) confidence levels before accepting a hypothesis, since the main aim is to ensure that falsehoods are not accepted into the body of knowledge. In regulating risk, however, the aim is to avoid harm, so to insist on this degree of certainty before taking precautions would seem negligent.[12] The problem is to decide *how far* in advance of certainty we should we act. Claim 2 may be read as suggesting a complete turning of the tables, prohibiting new technologies until their safety can be demonstrated with 95 per cent confidence. This, however, appears on the face of it equally unjustifiable, given that delaying or failing to implement a new technology may itself cause significant harms. There are of course numerous ways in which a balance between these two poles might be struck, but if the Precautionary Principle is to stand any chance of justifying a moratorium it must give higher priority to the *avoidance of new technological risks* than to the benefits, including the reduction of existing risks, that the new technology might bring.

Kristin Shrader-Frechette offers two arguments for this sort of prioritisation.[13] First, she claims that the kinds of risk associated with *implementing an unsafe technology* are typically more serious than those associated with *failing to implementing a safe one*. This is plausible for the kinds of technology she primarily has in mind, such as the chemical and nuclear technologies that produced catastrophic loss of life at Bhopal and Chernobyl, but does not seem applicable to the case of GM crops. In the case of herbicide tolerant and pest resistant crops, the alleged risks and benefits appear to be of similar kind and magnitude: an intensification on the one hand, or a reduction on the other, of the kinds of environmental impact already produced by conventional agriculture. Given the rough symmetry of these outcomes, and assuming genuine scientific uncertainty as to which will in fact occur, there would appear to be a good case for proceeding with field trials. The risk of some environmental damage around the trial locations would appear to be worth taking *if* there is a serious prospect that the crop in question will help to *reduce* such damage when planted on a wider scale.

The case for a *general* moratorium on GM crops was seen above to rest on the claim that GM crops may be less stable than conventional ones and hence have unpredictable and damaging effects. However, unless we are able give some concrete account of these effects and some reason for thinking that they will indeed occur, we will be unable to say whether they are sufficiently serious to outweigh the potential benefits of GM crops. The fact that unknown but very serious effects cannot be absolutely ruled out, is insufficient to justify a moratorium, since this would apply to any innovation whatsoever, and would leave us equally unable to rule out the possibility that *non-implementation* would be even more damaging. (For example, the ability to produce new crop varieties adapted to conditions such as drought more rapidly than is possible by conventional breeding techniques may prove crucial in a world where rapid and unpredictable climate change is widely anticipated.)

Shrader-Frechette's second argument for a precautionary approach rests on the idea (derived from medical ethics) that we have a right not to have risk imposed upon us without our free informed consent. One problem is that this appears over-restrictive, giving the most risk-averse members of society a veto over many public activities. But my main objection is to Shrader-Frechette's assumption that our rights are exclusively negative, and the act-omission distinction that this view embodies. For Shrader-Frechette we violate a person's rights by imposing risk on them, but not by omitting to provide them with the means of escaping risks that they already face. So, whereas Shrader-Frechette's first argument took the risks resulting from the implementation of an unsafe technology to be *materially* more serious than those resulting from the failure to implement a safe technology, the argument from negative rights and the act-omission distinction takes the former to be *morally* more serious even if the two are materially similar. This argument, however, is only as strong as the act-omission distinction on which it rests, and this distinction is not only controversial but also in tension with Shrader-Frechette's own aim of protecting the most vulnerable, since this frequently requires positive action to avert existing risks.

By contrast I would endorse the view, taken in the Nuffield report, that distributive justice requires us to give priority to meeting the most urgent needs of the worst off, even if that involves some risk to the less urgent interests of the better off.[14] Thus, a GM technology which held out a *serious* prospect of helping to feed the world's hungry, or preventing blindness due to vitamin-A deficiency, should be pursued even at some cost to the ability of the well-fed to enjoy a countryside rich in farmland wildlife. Where the Nuffield report goes wrong, in my view, is that, in a mirror image of environmentalists' indiscriminate opposition to GM crops, it too pays insufficient attention to the distinctions among them, and thus takes the possibility of alleviating hunger, and achieving other important benefits, to justify a 'moral imperative' to promote GM crops in general, rather than the specific avenues of research from which these benefits are likely to flow.

Conclusions

The arguments presented in this chapter support the following conclusions. Firstly, relevant distinctions should be drawn between different GM crops, rather than declaring blanket approval or a blanket moratorium. Secondly, since the risks highlighted by opponents of GM crops can apply also to new non-GM varieties, both should in principle be subject to the same case-by-case evaluation. And thirdly, in evaluating new varieties of either kind we should not seek to eliminate risk altogether but should exercise a degree of caution dependent on the relative importance of the risks and benefits of the particular crop, evaluated according to principles of distributive justice. Nothing in this chapter implies that the products currently being promoted by biotechnology companies should be embraced by environmentalists, but it does imply the need for a careful and balanced appraisal of the empirical evidence concerning their environmental effects, and for an open mind about the benefits, environmental and otherwise, that future developments in GM technology may bring.

Notes

1   Nuffield Council On Bioethics (1999) *Genetically Modified Crops: the Social and Ethical Issues,* London, Nuffield Council on Bioethics.
2   Nuffield Council, op. cit. §§6.20-6.22. Whether or not the particular claims made for current GM crops are true there seems to be no reason in principle why they should not produce benefits as well as risks for the environment.
3   E.g. Jeremy Rifkin (1998), 'Apocalypse when?', *New Scientist,* 31 October, p.36.
4   Nuffield Council, op. cit., p.148.
5   E.g. Greenpeace (2000) Food, The Environment, And Genetically Modified Organisms, http://www.greenpeace.org.uk/Multimedia/Live/FullReport/1222.PDF, p.2.
6   For related discussion see M. Häyry (1994) 'Categorical objections to genetic engineering – a critique' in A. Dyson and J. Harris (eds) *Ethics and Biotechnology,* London, Routledge.
7   Greenpeace spokespersons in a number of media interviews have appeared to take this view. See also the statement by Helen Wallace (Greenpeace Senior Scientist) in *New Scientist,* 14 August 1999, p.46, and Greenpeace, op. cit., p.1. The Nuffield report refers to such a view at op. cit. §6.41.
8   Friends of the Earth (1999) GMOs: the case for a moratorium, http://www.foe.co.uk/resource/reports/gmo_case_for_moratorium.html, October 1988, revised June 2001. The report also calls for a similar moratorium on the import of GM food and seeds and further patenting of genes, but these are beyond the scope of the present chapter.
9   The case of Pioneer Hi-Bred's Smart Canola oilseed rape is reported in *New Scientist,* 27 February 1999, p.4.
10   Nuffield Council, op. cit., §§6.16-6.17.
11   For discussions of the Precautionary Principle see T. O'Riordan and J. Cameron (eds) (1994) *Interpreting the Precautionary Principle,* London, Earthscan.
12   A similar view is taken by K. S. Shrader-Frechette (1991) *Risk and Rationality,* California, University of California Press, ch. 9.
13   The following is a fairly loose reconstruction of Shrader-Frechette's arguments in op. cit., ch. 9. She does not refer to the Precautionary Principle by name, but discusses the 'Producer Strategy' of prioritising the reduction of 'producer' or 'industry' risk over the reduction of 'consumer' or 'public' risk. These labels are misleading in that the benefits foregone by refusing new technologies need not accrue only to producers, as Shrader-Frechette's own discussion acknowledges.
14   Nuffield Council, op. cit., §§1.13, 1.27, 4.1-4.3.

Chapter 15

Everyday Risk and the Deliberate Release of Genetically Modified Crops

Shahrar Ali

The concept of risk and its related practices of risk assessment, risk management and risk perception, have found widespread currency in environmental policy. The two preceding chapters in this section have featured ethical and environmental issues raised by new genetic technologies when these are applied in the non-human living world. A central concern has been the issue of risk.

In the course of this chapter I attempt to sharpen our thought about risk by reviewing its relevance to everyday life. After considering the social response to more familiar technologies, I evaluate the central role of risk-related concepts in relation to policy on the deliberate release into the environment of genetically modified organisms. In the context of the controversy in Europe over GM crops, and in contrast to the spread such developments have typically enjoyed in the US, the precautionary outlook is defended as rationally responsible.[1]

Probability and magnitude

There are several ways of carving up the terrain with respect to our thought about risk. The Royal Society typifies risk as, 'The combination of the probability, or frequency, of occurrence of a defined hazard and the magnitude of the consequences of the occurrence.' 'Hazard' is identified as 'a property or situation that in particular circumstances could lead to harm' (Fairman, Mead and Williams, 1988, p.2).

This formulation classifies as risks the kind of uncertainties with respect to eventualities a human agent is likely to traffic in on a daily basis. There will be risks associated with simply leading a fairly unexceptional social existence in a modern liberal democracy, for instance. Travelling to and from work, aside from any particular risks associated with one's chosen vocation, are ways of accepting, more or less consciously, risks invariably attendant upon locomotion.

It may be that we choose not to think, or not to remind ourselves, about risks taken on a daily basis, or that we are psychologically disposed not to do so. It is an interesting question to what extent our focussing on particular risks and not others is dictated by a perception that some class of possible harms be recognised as normatively acceptable or simply inevitable.[2] A sense of this question should alert us to the fact that the type of risks of concern to environmental legislators is likely to relate to those perceived as hitherto unencountered, or issuing out of the development and introduction of new technologies. At the limit, then, even our estimation—or the estimation on our behalf by others—of those risks considered worthy of quantification and qualification is affected by a perception of what counts as normatively acceptable.

We can judge what risks count as going beyond the normatively acceptable in three distinct ways. Exposure to a hazardous material beyond one's control counts as an *involuntary* risk; consent on the part of those exposed may have been either assumed or neglected. The release of a microorganism into the environment, where irretrievability is at issue, counts as an *irreversible* risk; a former, supposedly safer state of affairs can no longer be returned to—permanently. And a *hidden* risk is one where it is not possible to see or comprehend the nature of the risk; it may require intuition, or specialisation, to make a tutored approximation of it.

The Royal Society definition speaks of the combination of (a) probability and (b) magnitude of a harm occurring. But it is precisely in determining these variables, and knowing how to combine or weight them, that the challenge of risk assessment lies.

It may not be rational in war, for example, ever to voluntarily initiate a nuclear exchange. But there is a quantifiable probability associated with the possibility of a nuclear weapon exploding accidentally. The possibility has been around ever since a nuclear weapon was assembled and its probability has increased with every additional weapon. Suppose the probability is as small as the chance of a jet aircraft colliding with your motor vehicle in your lifetime. Our perception of the gravity of attendant risk remains affected by an estimation of the magnitude of the consequence if it did occur. In the event of two chance occurrences equally improbable we regard the nuclear accident with greater aversion, where the damage to life and environment would be more extensive.[3]

Risk levels

The risk assessor typically tries to represent these two risk criteria, probability and harm's magnitude, as a single risk judgment. One author, David MacKenzie, follows a standard according to which judgments about risk are ordered along a continuum from low to high. MacKenzie uses these examples: (i) hang gliding is a *high* risk activity; (ii) an infrequent event with a large consequence, such as an earthquake on the east coast of the US counts as a *low* risk occurrence; (iii) an event that has never occurred in recorded history, such as a meteor striking the North American continent, has a *very low* risk; and (iv) a *mixed* risk would represent an increased frequency of events against a background of occurrences, such as additional cases of cancer beyond what is normally expected (Mackenzie, 1994).

Equivocation persists in how these two risk criteria are to be weighted in deriving a purported unitary judgment. Perhaps hang gliding counts as a high-risk activity because if one's wing collapsed one would be left with the unlively prospect of free falling to earth from a great height. But if it is the unpalatability of the outcome, when it occurs, that determines the level of risk, then, in all consistency, an earthquake on the east coast of the US quite arguably counts as a high risk event, too. It seems that MacKenzie equivocates in his examples between representing either probability or judgments of respective magnitudes as the criteria for arriving at a univocal gauge of the level of risk.

We should have anticipated this difficulty, for we seem to be seeking a rational means of combining two judgments that are strictly incommensurable. How might we combine a mathematical probability, supposing it available, with a measure of harm as undesired outcome? The probability is quantitative, and the harm, though it may be quantifiable in certain respects, is at base qualitative, providing us with a subjective—at best intersubjectively globally agreed upon—standard of what counts as worth avoiding or preventing. The qualitative judgment requires us to clarify, gauge and prioritise what counts as valuable in our lives; personally, socially and globally.

Estimation and acceptability

A distinction is sometimes advanced between the estimation and acceptability of a risk. MacKenzie treats the former—risk estimation—as the determination of a judgment as to the level of risk, supposedly a largely scientific question. Whereas the latter—risk acceptability—is considered a political question, concerning the priorities of the government of the day with respect to welfare expenditure or preventive health measures, for example. MacKenzie defends this picture of 'political reality' by averring that if the US spent as much for untimely death caused by smoking tobacco as she did on coal mine safety, there would not be any money left for any other purpose.

The sense in which political realism affects our acceptance of some policies over others fits into our characterisation of risk assessment as invariably taking place against a background of assumptions about what counts as normatively acceptable. This type of contextual consideration, however, may be more or less pervasive. The question of how to commit finite resources to managing risks which compete for those resources arguably presupposes a less pervasive form of normative judgment than does the question what counts as a risk deserving of attention in the first instance. Your taking some hazard to be too unpalatable to allow to happen will determine how much resource you, if in a position of political authority, would be prepared to allocate. Your political colleague may consider that same hazard to be quite acceptable; and whilst we may suppose either of your political strategies to diverge, that divergence is more accurately accounted for not as a difference in judgment as to the political acceptability of a risk but rather as a difference in estimate as to the nature of the risk that the hazard would bring.

So the distinction between estimating risks and judging them more or less politically acceptable is not so sharp as might have been hoped. Nor could the estimation of those risks be a wholly scientific enterprise. If what counts as scientific is exhausted by the application of currently described natural laws and principles—including mathematics—, how could sufficient allowance be made for the enterprise, inherently subjective at point of testimony, of gauging how much people care about preventing the occurrence of certain harms—the qualitative dimension of risk estimation? If what counted as scientific could be revised to include our best empirical generalisations concerning human behaviour and psychology, that might allow us to introduce more of the qualitative elements. Empirical and social observations do, in practice, make up a critical part of a risk assessor's initial data.

Probabilistic assessment

The risk assessor wishes to form a judgment that combines the probability of an event with its consequences. The consequences may be as difficult to determine as is the gauging of individuals' subjective reactions to harms occurring. Criteria are sometimes simpler; individuals running an insurance company can take the prospective harm to their business as determinable in solely economic terms. A standard procedure is to multiply the probability of an event by the amount of potential loss. The product is called the expectation of loss and may be used as a final measure of risk. An event which has one chance in ten thousand of happening and would cause a loss of fifty million Euros if it did, would make the expected loss five thousand Euros. That figure could form the basis of what the company charged as a premium.

Estimating probabilities associated with risk assessment can of course be complicated. The risk of engine failure in a civil aircraft may occur when several prior circumstances are met, or simply when fuel cuts out (though several factors may have conspired to give rise to that). A *fault tree* is the name given to a diagram constructed to enable us to trace the prospective paths that would lead to an unwanted outcome. An *event tree* is the inverse procedure, by which we take the outcome as initial event and trace the possible consequences. *Probabilistic risk assessment* is the method by which we combine the probabilities associated with either possible faults or possible consequences.

Three rules of probability are particularly important in risk assessment. The first allows us to calculate the probability with which two independent events may occur by *multiplying* the probability of each alone. The second rule allows us to determine, of two events that mutually exclude one another, the probability of either occurring as the *sum* of the probabilities of each alone. The third rule is a mathematical means for estimating the likely error, or give and take, that a probabilistic calculation entails. It is the *standard deviation*, or square-root-of-N rule, that tells us what for a given count, N, is the range across which that count would count as typical. If a striker scores 25 goals per season, on average, the standard deviation expected, the range between which the striker could be regarded as maintaining his form, would be 25 plus or minus five; that is, between 20 and 30 goals per season.

Risk management

H.W. Lewis, in *Technological Risk*, writes that, 'Management is what is done to limit risk, and assessment is what is done to determine whether the results are satisfactory. They tend to get mixed up' (Lewis, 1992, p.92). Clearly, assessment is what is done prior to the drawing up of managerial options, and perhaps that is why the demarcations tend to get 'mixed up'. After all, a good assessment will be conditioned by awareness of realistic practical strategies—current technology—as will a management strategy be dependent upon the compilation of relevant data; so the two operations are interrelated. And earlier in his monograph, Lewis outlines two basic strategies for the management of risk: prevention and mitigation.

Table 1: Risk in Four Fields of Technology

FIELD	EXAMPLE	RISK PROFILE	RISK MANAGEMENT
Toxic Chemicals	Methyl isocyanate, an intermediary in the production of pesticides	One hundred times more dangerous than cyanide gas, causes damage to respiratory tract and organs	Actual case, Bhopal (3 Dec 1984): gas leakage caused by exothermic reaction with water, killing 2,500, injuring thousands; investigation demonstrated a combination of human error, mechanical failure and managerial shortcomings
	Lead poisoning, accumulation in blood resulting from drinking water from lead-soldered pipes or inhaling exhaust emissions	Greater than 30 milligrams per decilitre in the blood causes symptoms such as personality change, headache and abdominal disorder	Curtailing or eliminating use of leaded gasolines and lead-soldering

Civil Aviation	Build redundancy into aircraft components to safeguard against single-point failures, e.g. multiple engines and instruments	Fatality rate for passengers one per billion passenger-miles, ten times better than average for automobiles	Actual case, Lockheed L-1011 (5 May 1983), all three engines disabled in turn due to independent oil leakages; pilot managed to restart one engine to avert crisis; investigation identified failure to install all three sets of engine oil O-rings correctly as cause; advice issued not to let same crew handle all elements of a redundant system
Ionising Radiation	Fission of uranium or plutonium isotopes to generate nuclear power results in radioactive fission fragments	Ionising radiation measured in roentgen equivalent man (rem); permitted exposure to nuclear workers 5,000 millirem per year; exposure over 400 rem kills 50% of persons exposed due to critical cell damage	Actual case, Chernobyl (April 1986), resulted from carrying out of a test regime with safety features fully disabled; cause of accident largely due to human error
Biotechnology	Genetically modified crops, e.g. Bt maize	Widespread uncertainty regarding possible harm from cross-pollination of GM pollen with wild crops; potential to damage both ingestors and biosphere irreversibly	Conduct limited, experimental field trials on new GM crops seeking market licences prior to any full-scale plantings; but do not such trials already effect changes to the gene pool?

Prevention lowers the probability of an unwanted event. Mitigation lowers the severity of the consequences that such an event would result in. A preventive measure, also regulatory, is the setting of a speed limit on highways with the intention of lowering the risk of road traffic accidents. What counts as a sufficient level of prevention, an acceptable level of risk? A world in which pedestrians had considerable safeguard from the possibility of being run over would be a world in which motor vehicles and cyclists did not exist, so it seems that some level of danger to pedestrians is regarded as an acceptable or inevitable part of modern life.

Mitigation describes the measures drawn up to deal with the accidental release of radioactive material from a nuclear power plant. Locals faced with radioactive release from the Chernobyl power plant in April 1986, for example, could have been advised either to evacuate immediately or to remain sheltered for a time before evacuating. Postponed evacuation had the advantage of limiting exposure to radioactive material with shorter half-lives, the strategy adopted by scientific advisers signalling to others their evacuation.

Technological fields in which the need for risk management has been widely recognised are: chemical toxins, civil aviation, ionising radiation and biotechnology. The table above takes examples from these fields.

Knowledge and consent

Incomplete knowledge renders risk assessment problematic. Our limitation as knowing subjects presents itself under both quantitative and qualitative dimensions of risk estimation.

Consider the difficulty of calculating probabilities. Is there always a determinate answer to a probabilistic question? If our best theory says not, because the system is inherently chaotic, then it makes less sense to attempt a measure of it. Take as another case the probability of an explosive accident, small yet greater than zero. A measure, though conceivable, may exceed our practical ability.

Where we can make calculations, qualitative deliberations may require considerable epistemic mastery, both with respect to initial risk estimation and subsequent risk acceptance. Suppose we have the ability to perfectly gauge our own evaluative reactions towards risk, and explicitly enough for the sake of policy considerations. But our ability to determine and weigh in the attitudes of others, for the sake of reaching wider consensus, is bound to be imperfect.

Drawing a distinction between knowledge and consent helps us to diagnose the implications for policy of quantifiable measures, subjective estimates and social acceptances of risk.

Read the table in the following way: Assume that two states of knowledge typify the impact of some technology, certitude or uncertainty, as entered under the first column. The next column represents four different states of consent to be had by or between one or more groups considering their attitudes to the technological impact in question. The last column diagnoses the likely character of future dialogue between two or more groups whose knowledge and consent bases vary along four different rows.

Table 2: Knowledge and Consent-Based Challenges to Risk

KNOWLEDGE	CONSENT	MANAGEMENT CHALLENGE
Certitude	Complete	Dialogue
	Disagreement	Differences perceived between parties in principle reconcilable
Uncertainty	Dependent on further knowledge	Try to increase knowledge
	Technology wholly unaccepted, independent of state of knowledge	Diagnosis: Disagreement likely to persist even after dialogue conducted in context of increasing information

Two patterns emerge. Under both the first and second rows, though consent between groups may be either complete or incomplete, whilst certitude obtains in respect of the impact of some technology, any outstanding disagreement is in principle reconcilable. Under the second row, where disagreement between groups about the desirability of a technology initially prevails, a managerial strategy may elect to focus on the groups' evaluative attitudes in prospective dialogue.

A further pattern, under both the third and fourth rows, reveals the endeavour to secure consent between groups compounded by the failure of certitude in respect of the technological impact initially. Under the third and fourth rows, either of which may represent positions in the GMO debate, knowledge claims are suspect. Where there is acceptance between the groups of shared technological goals, consent depends upon the pursuit of better knowledge. Where uncertainty coexists with the rejection by one party of the merit of pursuing the technology disagreement is likely to be intractable.

The Deliberate Release Directive

Since the 1980s public and political debate regarding the risks associated with the use of genetically modified organisms in commercial contexts has grown. Debating factions often assess risk in different ways. Attitudes can polarise between companies seeking advantage through the commercialisation of GM products and individuals with ethical qualms about the permissibility of modifying genes at all. Polarisation is widened when the conception of risk employed by either party is conditioned by implicit, often conflicting, ideas about those values most worth preserving or promoting; such ideas as the having of an economic goal against the living in accordance with tradition.

A more open debate—leaving open the question of how to determine risk— occurs between practitioners characterisable as equally scientific in outlook yet who differ over the knowledge base required by risk assessment. Molecular biologists have portrayed GM products as familiar, emphasising their predictability and inherent safety. Ecologists, to the contrary, have tended to regard the genetic novelty of GMOs as a source of environmental unpredictability, with the introduction of novel genes into a habitat uncontrolled relative to laboratory settings characterised as potentially hazardous.

Whereas the US regulatory structure has allowed development of GM products to proceed rapidly, nation states of the European Union have constructed special legislation and exercised considerable regulatory control. The European Community adopted Council Directive 90/220/EEC of 23 April 1990 on the deliberate release into the environment of genetically modified organisms. This provided a common framework for regulating releases of genetically modified organisms and served as a means of responding to key protagonists in the risk debate.[4]

The Preamble to the Deliberate Release Directive is unequivocally precautionary in content. It cites the requirement, under the Treaty, that Community action relating to the environment be based on the principle that *preventive* action be taken. It acknowledges that not only may living organisms released into the environment reproduce and cross national frontiers, thereby affecting other Member States, but that such effects of releases may be *irreversible*. It acknowledges that protection of human health and the environment require due attention to be given to the *control of risks* from deliberate releases. It distinguishes between organisms obtained through genetic techniques which have been conventionally used in a number of applications and have a *long safety record*, to which the Directive will not apply, and novel technologies. It highlights the importance of basing the provisions of Member States with respect to the functioning of the internal market on a *high level of health, safety, environmental and consumer protection*. It highlights the necessity of establishing harmonised procedures and criteria for the case-by-case evaluation of the *potential risks* arising from GMO releases such as: the carrying out of a case-by-case *environmental risk assessment prior to* a release; the adoption of release protocols that permit a subsequent increase in scale of a release *only if* the result of an evaluation at an immediately preceding step legitimates it on safety grounds; and the submission of a notification to the national competent authority by any person anticipating a deliberate release, where that notification contains a technical dossier of information including a full environmental risk assessment and *appropriate safety and emergency responses*.

In the general provisions of the Directive itself, the first article again asserts the objective of *protecting human health and the environment* within the framing of laws, regulations and administrative provisions of the Member States with respect to GMO releases. Member States are correspondingly obliged, under article 4, to ensure all appropriate measures be taken to *avoid adverse effects* on human health and the environment that might arise from a release; to designate the requisite competent authority responsible for carrying out the requirements of the Directive; and to ensure that this authority organises appropriate *control measures and inspections*.

The precautionary approach

We have noted how the Directive makes explicit use of terms such as *preventive action, environmental protection, control of risks, potential risk*, and *adverse effects*. The precautionary approach, in this framework, attempts to prevent hazards not yet documented for GMOs; in part, by determining what counts as insufficiently documented. It cannot be that novel GMO releases, due to their currency, could have established long safety records; therefore, under the condition of insufficiency, precaution should be adopted by default. In the absence, also, of quantifiable or certifiable risk profiles the precautionary outlook may be said to emphasise the qualitative dimension to risk.[5]

Regulatory attitudes to GMO releases have been subjected to further legislative scrutiny since February 1998, when the Commission presented a proposal for a European Parliament and Council Directive amending Directive 90/220/EC.[6] Whilst an account of legislation in this field at any one time risks becoming obsolete, due to the impact of intense revisionary activity, let us assume that our concern with prevailing attitudes to risk is not so subject to termly variation as might render this account unilluminating. The aim of the proposal is to make the procedure for granting consent to the placing on the market of GMOs more efficient and more transparent, to limit such consent to a fixed period (renewable) and to introduce compulsory monitoring after GMOs have been placed on the market. It also provides for a *common methodology to assess the risks associated* with the release of GMOs and a mechanism allowing the release of GMOs to be modified, suspended or terminated where new information becomes available on the risks of such release. The main thrust of the revisionary proposals is to maintain and bolster the explicit objective of the original Directive, to protect human health and the environment.

Recognition of, and political reaction to, the proposed amendments is dramatised in two Declarations reached by a Ministerial Meeting of the Environmental Council of the EU on 24/25 June 1999, in Luxembourg, which evidence a systematic magnification of risk cognates given currency in the original Directive. With abstentions from France, Ireland and Italy, delegations from Austria, Belgium, Denmark, Finland, Germany, Greece, Italy, Luxembourg, the Netherlands, Spain, Sweden, and the UK reached agreement on the need for *additional procedures* for the renewal of consents and the handling of consents given under the pre-existing Directive, and for the monitoring and handling of new information and objections to GMOs which have already received consents.[7]

Whereas the original Directive indicated consultation with the public to be left at the *discretion* of the Member State leading the regulation of a given notification, the Declarations of the Council submit that consultation be made *mandatory* in order to *restore public and market confidence* and *restore the trust of public opinion*. The Declarations also magnify the conditions on what would count as an adequate risk assessment by emphasising both *transparency* and importing the concepts, respectively, of *tightness* and *strictness* into the regulatory regimes. In addition, the first Declaration requests that no *adverse effects* (a tool of the original Directive) be precisely *demonstrated*.[8] Until such condition is met, Member State signatories will not authorise marketable GMOs. The language of the second Declaration is perhaps more preventive still, asserting that, in absence of such Commission rules governing traceability and labelling of GMOs, new authorisations for growing and market placement *will be suspended*.

Summary conclusion

We characterised the two criteria that enter into the determination of a risk as the probability of a harm's occurring and the severity of the harm if it does occur. We acknowledged that our risk attitudes are conditioned by the normative background against which such judgments are perceived as acceptable or not. We acknowledged that a sharp distinction between estimation and acceptability cannot be sustained. We registered the potential, and limitations, of probabilistic reasoning in the determination of judgments where knowledge bases are incomplete and evaluative assumptions contested. Controversy over the potential benefits and harms of releasing genetically modified organisms into the environment were diagnosed in terms of limitations in knowledge and consent.

The precautionary outlook of the Deliberate Release Directive has been explicated in relation to the EU's objective of protecting human health and the environment. More recent political initiatives have reinforced and bolstered the precautionary approach in order to restore public confidence. Are these precautionary attitudes justified?

Our review of the topic of risk invites us to endorse the precautionary attitude as the rationally responsible policy on a number of grounds. First, the risks associated with GM products are not normatively familiar: the release of a novel gene into the environment is irreversible and the mechanisms by which gene transference occur are neither visible to the naked eye, readily traceable nor under our direct control. Second, even if knowledge were complete, the aim of environmental policy is not exhausted by the agenda of science. A policy at once subjecting itself to a highly democratised process, that remains sensitive to complex long-term considerations, does non-accidentally direct us to the rationally superior result.[9]

Notes

1   This chapter is based on work I undertook as a Research Scholar in the Science and Technology Options Assessment Unit of the European Parliament, Luxembourg in 1999. I thank Dick Holdsworth and David Bowe MEP for stimulating dialogue, Josefine for invigoration, Oliver Schick for proofreading, and the editors to this volume.

　　Though I do not undertake to argue this point, the reader will notice that my characterisation of the precautionary outlook as rationally responsible invites a somewhat stronger interpretation than that defended by Jonathan Hughes in the preceding chapter to this volume. In debate with him at the Society for Applied Philosophy Conference 2000, I have said that the risks associated with GMOs differ in degree from everyday risks to an extent that justifies their being treated as different in kind and not consistent with all the degrees of caution (or permissibility) he wishes to advance.

2   The day following the Gonesse Concorde crash, in dialogue with a BBC correspondent, a French Aviation Authority official was asked, 'So we have to live with the risk of death?', to which he replied, 'It's hard to say this today, but [yes] this is our life'. The contention here seems to be that we reconcile ourselves to the prospect of near certain fatality following a certain type of free fall crash because we do not wish to dispense with the technological conveniences of life. I suspect, however, that we choose not to remind ourselves about the severity of the consequence in this case. [*Newsnight*, 26 July 2000]

3   Recall the eloquent expression of Bertrand Russell's pacifistic sentiments. In an exchange of letters with Lord Gladwyn in 1964, he writes: '[I]t is a simple matter of mathematical statistics that the more nuclear missiles there are the greater is the danger of nuclear accident. Vast numbers of rockets and other missiles, primed for release and dependent upon mechanical systems and slight margins in time, are highly subject to accident . . . In estimating the wisdom of a policy, it is necessary to consider not only the possibility of a bad result, but also the degree of badness of the result. The extermination of the human race is the worst possible result, and even if the probability of its occurring is small, its disastrousness should be a deterrent to any policy which allows of it', in Russell, Bertrand (2000 ed.) *Autobiography,* Routledge, p.695 ff.

4   Directive 90/220/EEC on the Deliberate Release into the Environment of Genetically Modified Organisms, *Official Journal of the European Communities,* L117 08.05.1990. The Directive consists of 24 Articles, spread across four distinct parts—part A dealing with general provisions, part B with non-market-oriented releases, part C with marketable products, and part D with final provisions—followed by three Annexes.

5   Some researchers have contended that the best way of thinking about a precautionary policy with respect to GMOs is as 'uncertainty-based regulation'. R. von Schomberg, for example, argues for a shift in legislative emphasis from the '(impossible) identification of quantifiable risk to the acceptability [or not] of uncertainties'. L. Levidow et al emphasise interpretative disparities across Member States as a way of revealing uncertainties: France, for example, associates risk with genetic imprecision and the UK ascribes to genetic novelty an 'inherent uncertainty'. See R. von Schomberg (1998), *An Appraisal of the Working in Practice of Directive 90/220/EC,* European Parliament, Brussels, Luxembourg and Strasbourg and L. Levidow et al (1998), *Environmental Risk Disharmonies of European Biotechnology Regulation,* 1999 hypertext document: binas.unido.org/binas/Library/cabi/levidow.html

6   COM(98)0085final 98/0072(COD), *Official Journal of the European Communities,* C139, 04.05.1998. The legislative, and inherently political, mechanisms of the European Institutes—the Parliament, the Commission and the Environmental Council—are complex and time-consuming, typified by the tabling of amendments and the convening of readings, secondary readings and co-decision procedures. By July 2000, the legislative revisions had not come into force, but were reaching their finality. In the interim, moratoria had been adopted by the majority of Member States.

7   Document of the 2194th Council Meeting, Luxembourg, Public Register of Council of the European Union Documents: ue.eu.int. Two Declarations were signed, the first by Denmark, Greece, Italy, Luxembourg and the UK; the second by Austria, Belgium, Finland, Germany, the Netherlands, Spain and Sweden.

8   Can it but be assumed that absence of evidence *demonstrates* evidence of absence?

9   For further evaluation of the Directive, legislative developments, and critical comparison of risk assessment in other EU policy areas, notably, the human exposure risk from BSE, and the risks posed by 4-MTA, endocrine-disrupting chemicals, and ionising radiation, see Ali, M.S. (1999), *Risk Assessment in EU Policy: Quantitative and Qualitative Aspects,* European Parliament, Brussels, Luxembourg and Strasbourg. It is interesting to note, for example, that in legislation on BSE a *worse-case assumption* is substituted for the determination of risk, where information is assumed otherwise inadequate.

References

Ali, M.S. (1999), *Risk Assessment in EU Policy: Quantitative and Qualitative Aspects,* European Parliament, Brussels, Luxembourg and Strasbourg.

COM(98)0085final 98/0072(COD), *Official Journal of the European Communities,* C139, 04.05.1998.

Directive 90/220/EEC on the Deliberate Release into the Environment of Genetically Modified Organisms, *Official Journal of the European Communities,* L117 08.05.1990.

Document of the 2194th Council Meeting, Luxembourg, Public Register of Council of the European Union Documents: ue.eu.int

Fairman, Mead and Williams (1998), *Environmental Risk Assessment: Approaches, Experiences and Information Sources,* European Environmental Agency, Copenhagen.

Levidow, L. et al. (1998), *Environmental Risk Disharmonies of European Biotechnology Regulation,* 1999 hypertext document:
binas.unido.org/binas/Library/cabi/levidow.html

Lewis, H.W. (1992), *Technological Risk,* Norton.

Mackenzie, David (1994), *Environmental Risk Analysis,* 1999 hypertext document:
binas.unido.org/binas/Library/book/mackenzie.html

Russell, Bertrand (2000 ed.) *Autobiography,* Routledge.

von Schomberg, R. (1998), *An Appraisal of the Working in Practice of Directive 90/220/EC,* European Parliament, Brussels, Luxembourg and Strasbourg.

Chapter 16

Public Deliberation and Private Choice in Human Genetics[1]

Michael Parker

It is clear from the earlier chapters in this volume that the continuing development of human genetics raises a wide variety of important ethical questions for us all, whether as healthcare professionals, patients, members of families or as individuals. A British Medical Association publication recently described human genetics as,

> a science characterised by rapid and spectacular advances in knowledge. The advances affect not only individual patients, but potentially society at large. Genetics opens possibilities to influence the composition of future generations and the sort of people brought into the world. It raises questions about human identity and free will. Speculation and research about how genes might predispose an individual to develop certain characteristics have long gone beyond the medical preoccupation with health and disease. The intriguing prospect of the heredity of character and behaviour such as criminality is increasingly debated. Human cloning or the possibility of parents selecting the intelligence quotient or other traits of their children appear to bring to life the cliché of 'man playing God' (British Medical Association, 1998).

As several of the authors contributing to this book have suggested, many of the ethical questions raised by genetics are not new but are given a new, more urgent, intensity by its development. Genetics raises difficult questions both in relation to ourselves and to those around us: to our patients, our families and communities, to other, more distant people, to future generations, and to the non-human world. In this concluding chapter I shall concentrate on the ethical issues arising in *human* genetics. An example of this which seems certain to be of increasing importance in the future is the question of the use of genetics in reproductive choice. The need to make decisions about public policy in this area combined with the interpersonal dimension of genetic information means that genetics also raises important questions about the relationship between the public and the private. When, for example, are my reproductive choices, if ever, a matter for me and my family, to be made in the privacy of our own home, and when are they, again if ever, a matter for public decision-making? In some ways genetics, particularly when combined with new reproductive technology, has forced the private into the public arena.[2]

The challenge posed by genetics is further intensified by the fact that despite widespread agreement about the problematic nature of the New Genetics, there is little consensus about the grounds upon which the ethical questions it raises should be addressed. To a certain degree, this is a reflection of a broader sense in which we live in a world that at the level of morality is deeply fragmented. For, it is something of a truism to say that,

> Under modern conditions of life none of the various rival traditions can claim prima facie general validity any longer. Even in answering questions of direct practical relevance, convincing reasons can no longer appeal to the authority of unquestioned traditions (Habermas, 1993).

How then, given this apparent lack of consensus and, given that the development and use of the New Genetics has implications and effects that range from those affecting families and individuals to those of global proportions, are we to go about making ethical decisions about its future development and use?

Patient-centred medicine in the community

It is common in the context of modern 'patient-centred' medicine, to argue that at the heart of any attempt to identify an ethical approach to medicine and to medical research must lie a commitment to the belief that, at least *prima facie*, people ought to be free to decide for themselves about the kinds of treatments or tests they receive and the information they wish to divulge, or to have divulged about them by healthcare professionals. It is widely accepted that this ought not always to be the case, that there will be times when a patient will not be competent to make such choices, and circumstances in which the competent autonomous choices of individuals will conflict with the interests of others. Nevertheless, it is widely accepted that the practice of ethical medicine requires us to take seriously the choices, wishes and desires of the patients we treat. This is often expressed as a requirement that practitioners and researchers respect the 'principle of autonomy' (Beauchamp et al., 1994).

This emphasis on autonomy and patient-choice in medicine has however in recent years been subjected to a certain amount of criticism, by feminists (Frazer et al., 1993) and by those who have come to be known as 'communitarians' (Lindemann Nelson et al., 1995), for being overly 'individualistic'. Communitarians for example, argue that there is a conflict in health care between the individualistic values that underlie patient-centred medicine and the communitarian values that sustain families and communities. Modern medicine's overriding focus on the benefit of the individual patient, they argue, has led to an unhealthy imbalance between individual and community values. They claim that when faced with conflicting treatment choices practitioners, policy makers and indeed patients themselves often adopt the individualistic values of the medical world leading them in their pursuit of individualism to undermine the values that sustain the families, relationships and communities in which they live.[3] The critics of personal autonomy argue moreover, that individualism fails to recognise that many of the most important ethical questions raised by modern medicine and elsewhere only arise at all because we are located in relationships and families and live in a world with others -a world that cannot be characterised in individual terms (Sandel, 1982). This means, they argue, that there is an important sense in which the moral questions posed by medicine can only be grasped at all in the light of a sense of our location in a world with others.

If these claims are valid with respect to medicine in general, they will be particularly so in relation to the question of whether patient-centred medicine can provide the basis for answers to the ethical questions raised by genetics. For this is where the tensions between individuals, their families and communities are likely to be at their most intense. If these claims are valid they pose a serious threat to patient-centred approaches to the new genetics. But are they valid?

Whilst each of these claims is important, they do not as they stand provide as powerful an argument for the rejection of 'patient-centredness' in healthcare as might at first appear to be the case. There are two quite different types of argument that might be used against the communitarian in this regard. The first of these arguments suggests that the communitarian critique of the 'individualism' of patient-centred medicine is based upon mistaken claims about the nature of patient choices and about the values by which they are informed. The second argument suggests that *contra* the claims of the communitarian, the concept of patient-centred medicine is in its own right deeply communitarian (Parker, 1999). If so, and if we are serious about communities and relationships, we ought to place more emphasis on personal autonomy rather than less.

The communitarian claim that an emphasis on autonomy is *necessarily* individualistic and anti-communitarian is plainly false. To advocate an approach to ethical decision-making based in the choices of individuals does not exclude the possibility that the values and choices of such individuals might have a social dimension (Kymlicka, 1991). Even if I am free to choose as an individual on the basis of my own values and desires, my choices may well turn out to be deeply communitarian in orientation. I may decide to spend more time with my family, to work with the homeless, to help the elderly or to donate my kidney to someone who needs it. Furthermore, in making my autonomous choices I may very well seek the opinions and suggestions of others. My choices need not necessarily be either selfish or detached. As an individual I might value my relationships with others very much indeed and even see them as a priority. It is not necessarily the case therefore that to call for an emphasis on individual autonomy is to advocate a 'socially unencumbered' approach to ethics (Sandel, 1982). Given the invalidity of this conceptual claim, the validity of the communitarian critique of the individualism of patient-centred medicine ultimately comes down to an empirical claim about the actual choices of real people and there seems little evidence to suggest that we are oblivious to communitarian concerns in our actual decision making. Indeed, the very fact that we express such concern about 'individualism' shows that we are in fact the holders of highly communitarian values. The implication of this is that private autonomous choices will not necessarily, or even contingently, fail to have a communal or public dimension.

I believe that we can go further than this negative claim however to argue that a genuine commitment to personal autonomy *requires* us to take human relationships very seriously. For, a moral and political emphasis on the value of autonomous decisions and on the promotion of autonomy implies a commitment not simply to freedom of choice for individual people but also to particular ways of living and deciding with others (Rousseau, 1968). To emphasise the value of patient choice and autonomy consistently is also to place particular value and emphasis upon certain forms of community and of communal life. To live a life that is truly one's own and genuinely autonomous is necessarily more than simply a matter of making choices on one's own and in one's own interest. We live in a world with other people, in networks of relationships, families and 'communities', and this means that to live an autonomous life is necessarily to engage in and to take seriously the social dimensions of and limitations on, one's choices and actions. There are at least three reasons for this. Firstly, we cannot be fully autonomous unless we have some say in the social world in which we live out our lives. It is only by such engagement that we can shape the world in which our choices occur and are made possible (Cohen et al., 1983). Secondly, it is by engaging with those around us and by making such choices that we develop our autonomy (MacIntyre, 1999). Personal autonomy is made possible by social interaction and in decision-making with others. It is not a skill that can be developed alone (Rousseau, 1968). Thirdly, communitarians are correct, it seems to me, in their claim that the very meaningfulness both of the concept of moral choice and of the moral dimension of the world in which we live out our lives, each of which is crucial to the autonomous life, is made possible by virtue of our location in a social world in which there is the use of moral concepts in moral discussion and argument and the use of reasons to justify moral positions (MacIntyre, 1999).

What these claims imply, if we accept them, is that a serious adherence to the value of autonomy is in many ways itself a deeply 'communitarian' position to adopt. This is because to argue consistently and seriously for the encouragement and expression of personal autonomy in patient-centred medicine is inevitably to support an enriched view of such autonomy and hence of patient-centredness.

Nevertheless, no coherent ethical approach to decision-making can rely *solely* on community-based values. Communitarians have rightly been criticised for their unjustifiably optimistic interpretation of community life and for their reliance on a much greater social coherence and sharing of values than actually exists (Parker, 1996). It seems empirically at least to be undesirable that many paradigmatic communitarian communities, such as the family, are as often sites of conflict, violence and clashes of values as they are of mutual support and shared values. It seems undeniable too that communitarians are also at the very least guilty of underplaying the potentially damaging effects of communities and of social pressure upon individuals and minority groups.[4]

Conflicts of values and the existence of disadvantage in real communities and families are problematic for communitarians because they emphasise that whilst communitarians describe very well the damage that can occur when people attempt to escape or are excluded from communities, they are incapable of explaining the damage that is sometimes caused by such 'communities' themselves. Some crucial dimensions of our moral world, notably the need to uphold the rights of individuals (say of the genetically disadvantaged) against the community at large are not consistent with a communitarian framework. Consequently communitarianism says little for those who feel themselves to be excluded from or at the fringes of communities because it fails to see that the convergence of ideas with those of the community is in itself no guarantee of justice. Ultimately, taken to its logical extreme the communitarian belief that the community, relationships and traditions are the highest goods, is also capable of justifying the oppression of minorities (including individuals) by the majority. Developments in testing and screening offered by the New Genetics offer the potential at least for just this kind of discrimination and this ought to make us particularly wary of the use of *overly* community-based approaches to decision-making in the case of the application or otherwise of the New Genetics. Whilst communitarians attack the emphasis on personal autonomy for its inability to recognise the fact that our understanding of moral problems arises out of our shared ways of life with others, communitarianism itself seems to lose sight of what is surely the central achievement of patient centred medicine which is the recognition that we need to be able to uphold the rights of individuals. Whilst the communitarian might reply that the good life can only be lived in a community wherein rights and responsibilities cohabit in a state of 'healthy balance' (Etzioni, 1994), this leaves dangerously open the question of just who is to decide the parameters of such a balance?

Public reason for personal autonomy

Any consistent approach to the making of ethical decisions in genetics must be capable of recognising the moral status of individual people and of their choices. An approach that is serious about autonomy must at the same time be capable of capturing the importance of both the communitarian conditions for the development of personal autonomy and of the communitarian dimension of the world in which we live. I want now briefly to sketch out some of the implications of these claims for ethical decision making in health care practice .

   In the context of a relatively abstract discussion about the relationship between individuals, relationships and communities in medical ethics, it is sometimes easy to overlook the fact that the individual and the community meet in the everyday relationships between real people. It is here, in the relationships between people, that the community comes to have an effect upon the lives of individuals and also here that individuals come to have an effect upon the communities in which they live (Parker, 1995). It follows from this and from the arguments I sketched out earlier in this paper that what is required if we are to make ethical choices about the future of human genetics (or indeed about any other ethically problematic area of health care practice), is a coherent interpersonal process of public reason and justification oriented towards the support and development of personal autonomy. For it is only within the context of a public process of this kind that it is possible to approach ethical decision-making in healthcare in a way which captures the value of both individuals and communities.

Such an approach, whilst in an important sense 'communitarian', is able to avoid the usual dangers of communitarianism because it is founded upon, and oriented towards, the development and exercise of personal autonomy. It differs from communitarianism also because the orientation of the process is not towards the support of values that sustain families and communities *per se*, but towards the development of communal processes and institutions only insofar as, and because, these processes and institutions promote and sustain the personal autonomy and the self-realisation of their members. This has the added advantage of providing room for a critique of those social and communal practices which do not promote or respect personal autonomy (such as infibulation).

A process of this kind, based as it is in a respect for and the promotion of personal autonomy would have to accord with certain principles, the justification of which would lie in the extent to which they too support or contribute to the actual expression and development of such autonomy and the extent to which they frame a process which facilitates such development. What would be the key features of such an approach?

Firstly, it follows from the emphasis on the value of personal autonomy that ethical decisions in genetics are best made, and in fact might in some cases only be capable of being made, by those people most likely to be affected by the decision at hand and this is to suggest that such a process would be one adhering to a *prima facie* principle of respect for 'personal autonomy'. Secondly, such an approach is also, for the same reason, one which emphasises 'participation' and this means that the requirement for decisions to be made by those most likely to be affected will in each case need to be assessed against a responsibility to ensure the participation of all who have a legitimate interest. This is to suggest that in practice decision-making will have to take a range of different interdependent forms, the form most appropriate in relation to any particular question being dependent upon the extent of legitimate interest in the question at hand. In the case of issues of widespread public or even global concern such as the genetic modification of crops, the sale of genetically modified foods or the funding of research into the development of new techniques such as reproductive cloning (Bulletin of Medical Ethics, 1999), for example, the most appropriate deliberative process might be publicly-funded consensus conferences or other deliberative decision-making models such as deliberative opinion polls (Fishkin, 1995) or appropriately constituted ethics committees. The principle of respect for 'personal autonomy' (in the broad sense outlined earlier) will mean however, that in some, perhaps most, instances decision-making will devolve to deliberative processes on a smaller scale such as those involving practitioners, patients and their families. And, given the underlying commitment of this approach to the development of personal autonomy, it will be perfectly appropriate, in many circumstances, for such deliberation to be the concern of the patient alone. Indeed, given the commitment of this approach to an enriched view of personal autonomy the default position in any decision will be that of the autonomy of the patient. Justification of the expansion of the process, in accordance with the principle of 'participation' to include others such as other family members or communities will depend upon the giving of reasons which cannot reasonably be rejected and which are commensurate with respect for personal autonomy.

The balance between the principles of respect for 'enriched personal autonomy' and 'participation' would inevitably in many cases be problematic, raising for example important questions about the relationship between the private and the public in ethical decision-making. This can be seen in many ways however as an opportunity. For, within this framework the question of the balance between participation and autonomy, and, the public and the private, would itself have to be resolved by appropriate processes of public deliberation oriented towards the encouragement of personal autonomy. Such a process (or processes) would enable us to address many of the most fundamental and difficult questions raised by the New Genetics. It may be perfectly reasonable for a community to decide, for example, through an appropriate process of deliberation, that certain reproductive choices are a matter for couples and individuals themselves to make 'in private' whilst considering others to be a matter for public consideration and assessment, on the grounds that there is a legitimate public interest in the question at hand (such interest being itself only justifiable in terms of the protection and promotion of the autonomy of its members).

One possible example in the arena of genetics and reproduction is the question of the right of couples to use genetic techniques to select the sex of their child.[5] At present such practices are illegal in the United Kingdom other than for the avoidance of sex-linked disorder. It is possible to imagine a deliberative process of the kind I have described coming to a different conclusion. It might for example be concluded that sex selection should neither be banned outright nor left to couples to decide for themselves. It might, for example, be agreed that some reasons for wanting to select the sex of ones child are valid whereas others are not. There might be no good reason to refuse sex selection in some circumstances, such as for example in the case of a couple who have a high probability of passing on a harmful sex-linked mutation to their child. At the other end of the spectrum it might be agreed that the selection of the sex of ones child on the basis of the social status of the children of a particular gender is unacceptable. One might imagine this being justified on the grounds that such practices are not compatible with a health care system oriented to the respect for and the development of enriched personal autonomy. Between these extremes there would be many other less clear-cut cases in which the giving of convincing reasons in the appropriate forum would be the key to whether or not the practice ought to be allowed. The default position in each case would be respect for the autonomy of the couple and the responsibility for justification will always lie with those who wish to override such autonomy, and not on the couple to justify why they wish to proceed. In practice of course such a system might be impossible to manage on a case by case basis and 'good practice guidelines' might have to be developed (by a similar process of deliberation) to cover all but the most exceptional of cases.

Conclusion

Developments in the New Genetics confront us with the most profound and difficult of moral choices. In the not too distant future, it may be appropriate for many of these choices to be considered a matter of personal or local concern. At this stage however, the future of genetic research and the development of novel treatments and techniques are rightly a matter of public concern and require public deliberation. The global dimension of much of this research and its implications requires that such deliberation ought often to have an international dimension. In a world in which there is much diversity of values and attitudes towards such questions it will inevitably be difficult to find common ground upon which to address them. For this reason I have argued that the resolution of many of the most important ethical questions raised by genetics, and in particular those that arise in relation to families, partnerships, relationships and communities, demands a deliberative and collective process of decision-making and I have sketched some of the features of such a process.

I have argued that, despite fundamental differences of values and disagreement about priciples, it is possible, based upon the shared sense we have that any solution to these problems will be one in which the choices, wishes and desires of individual people will be taken seriously, to build an effective and ethical decision-making process which also takes seriously the communal dimension of such questions. Whilst I have argued that such decision-making ought to adhere to these principles and ought in addition to have as its orientation the development of personal autonomy, such an approach will inevitably take a variety of forms and I have also described some of these in the paper. It is not possible however to specify these in the abstract because their formation and their acceptance will itself be dependent upon their origin in a deliberative process. Nevertheless, it is clear that such a range will stretch from extensive and wide-scale processes of public deliberation on issues such as the genetic modification of crops and of the development of germ line therapies, to decisions within families and couples and by individuals about certain kinds of genetic tests, reproductive choices and the sharing of personal genetic information. A deliberative process of the kind I have described offers the possibility of a resolution of some of these questions without itself depending upon an extensive set of deeply shared values, or the imposition of individualistic or communitarian principles. Nevertheless, whilst it does not itself depend upon a non-existent consensus, it offers the possibility of a developing, emerging consensus in a context of diversity -and thereby of addressing the third part of the problem with which I began this chapter, notably the existence of a disabling social fragmentation at the moral level. For, the building of deliberative processes of this kind has the added benefit of leading to the development of shared and relatively stable decision-making institutions, perhaps of increasingly shared values and is in this sense a deeply communitarian project (Edgar, 1999). Its value being too that it does not have built into it either a requirement, or even an aim, that we should reach general agreement or achieve the end of diversity. Rather, on the contrary, this is a process and an approach that suggests that such diversity of values is to some extent a condition for the possibility of an ethical decision-making process. Interestingly too, it suggests that if we are serious about the importance of relationships and about communities in ethical medicine we will take the principle of respect for personal autonomy, broadly conceived, very seriously indeed.[6]

Notes

1   A version of this chapter appeared in the Journal of Medical Ethics, 2000, Vol. 26:3. I would like to thank the publishers and the Editor of the JME for permission to reprint this paper here.

2   See for example a recent discussion of the consequences of the incorporation of European Human Rights legislation into UK law on the regulation of reproduction in The *Guardian Newspaper*: Monday 14th February, 2000: pages 1 and 3. Note in particular the comments both of Ruth Deech who is the Head of the Human Fertilisation and Embryology Authority and of Lady Warnock who chaired the 1984 committee of inquiry into human fertilisation and embryology.

3   See for example the case study with which Lindemann Nelson, H. and Lindemann Nelson, J. (1995) open their book *The Patient in the Family: an ethics of Medicine and Families.* New York, Routledge.

4   The experiences of Mental Health Service Users might be seen as a particularly important example of this; for this experience has often been one both of exclusion, discrimination and even of violence. See, Lindow, V. (1999) 'The Exclusion of Health Service Users' in M.Parker, *Ethics and Community in the Health Care Professions.* London, Routledge, pp.154-171.

5   I would like to thank Julian Savulescu and Justin Oakley for suggesting this example.

6   I would like to acknowledge of the support of a University of Melbourne Visiting Research Fellowship in summer 1999 during which I wrote this paper. I would also like to acknowledge the very insightful and useful comments made by Tony Hope, Richard Ashcroft and Julian Savulescu during the writing of this paper.

References

Beauchamp, T. and Childress, J. (1994), *Principles of Biomedical Ethics* (Fourth Edition), Oxford, Oxford University Press.

British Medical Association (1998), *Human Genetics*, London, British Medical Association, vol.1.

Special Issue of the Bulletin of Medical Ethics including several papers focusing on the proposed revision of the Helsinki Declaration and Medical Research in a global context, *Bulletin of Medical Ethics*, August 1999, Issue 150.

Cohen, J. and Rogers, J. (1983), 'Democracy' in *On Democracy: Toward a Transformation of American Society*, New York, Penguin.

Edgar, A. (1999), 'The Health Service as Civil Association', in M. Parker, *Ethics and Community in the Health Care Professions*, London, Routledge, pp.15-46.

Etzioni, A. (1994), *The Spirit of Community: The Reinvention of American Society*, London, Harper Collins.

Fishkin, J.S. (1995), 'The Deliberative Poll: Bringing Deliberation to Democracy', in *The Voice of the People*, Newhaven, Yale University Press, pp.161-181.

Frazer, E and Lacey, N. (1993), *The Politics of Community: A Feminist Critique of the Liberal-Communitarian Debate*, Hemel Hemstead, Prentice Hall, Europe.

Habermas J. (1993), *Justification and Application: Remarks on Discourse Ethics*, Oxford, Polity, p.151.

Kymlicka, W (1991), *Liberalism, Community and Culture*. Oxford, Oxford University Press.

Lindemann Nelson, H and Lindemann Nelson J. (1995) *The Patient in the Family*, New York, Routledge.

MacIntyre, A. (1999), *Dependent Rational Animals: Why Human Beings Need the Virtues*, London, Duckworth.

Parker, M. (1995), *The Growth of Understanding*, Aldershot, Ashgate.

Parker, M. (1996), 'Communitarianism and its Problems', in *Cogito*, November, pp.204-209.

Parker, M. (1999), *Ethics and Community in the Health Care Professions*, London, Routledge.

Rousseau, J.J. (1968), *The Social Contract or Principles of Political Right*, London, Penguin Books, pp.49-69.

Sandel, M. (1982), *Liberalism and the Limits of Justice*, Cambridge, Cambridge University Press, p.179.

Index